INNER ARTS 1

EXERCISES FOR KUNDALINI, AWAKENING AND SOVEREIGNTY

By Jana Dixon

AWAKENING SOVEREIGNTY SERIES 1

© Copyright 2019 Jana Dixon
Published by Amazon KDP

Second Edition
ISBN-13: 978-1-7336664-1-1

> "There is a celestial mind force,
> a great sympathetic force
> which is life itself,
> of which everything is
> composed."
> ~ John Worrell Keely

http://biologyofkundalini.com
http://jana-sovereignstate.blogspot.com
https://biologyofkundalini.academia.edu/JanaDixon

CONTENTS

CONTENTS iii
INTRODUCTION ix
CHAPTER 1: THE INNER ARTS 1
   Inner Dimensional Journey 2
   The Kinesthetic Innerceptive Senses 2
   Phi Transfiguration 3

CHAPTER 2: FOUNDATION INNER SKILLS 5
   • Stopping 5
   • Make Like a Rock 5
   • Inner Smile 6
   • The Three Kings 7
   • Dropping the Tongue (Off Switch) 8
   • Plugging Into The Sovereign State 8
   • Grounding = Harmonizing 9
   • Establishing The Mind's Eye 9
   • Toning 9
   • Syncopated Toning 10
   • Getting a Grip on the Brainstem 10
   • Opening The Mouth of God 11
   • Noble Seat 11
   • Belly Love 12
   • Relaxation Response 12
   • Dance 12
   • Sungazing 12
   • Moon Gazing 13
   • Eliminating Enervation 14
   • Ileocecal Valve 14
   Meditation and Neuro-Enhancement 15
   Rooting the Prefrontals 16
   Clearing the Attic 16
   Advanced Human Character Traits 17
   Wholebrain Gama Wave 18
   Plugging In 20
   Holy-Healing-Wholing 22

CHAPTER 3: MASTER SOVEREIGNTY SERIES 24
   • Cardiomuscular Release (CMR) 25
   • Psychospacial Meditation 27
   • Heart-Tree Meditation 29
   • Heart-Eyes Meditation 31
   • The Fount of Happiness 31
   • Happy Hippocampus Meditation 32
   • Hypothalamus Assurance Boost 32

- Goodifying Emeditation 33
- Neuroemotional Reprogramming 34
- Primal Release Pose 38
- The Inner Candle Meditation 40
- Complex Inner Candle Meditation.. 41
- The Reptile and the Butterfly 41
THE URAEUS 42
- Uraeus Meditation 44
The Kabala and the Egg... 47

CHAPTER 4: PRINCIPLE SOVEREIGNTY PRACTICES 49
- Light Sword Meditation.. 49
- Light Sword and Uraeus Meditation Combo 50
- Blue Spot Meditation... 50
- Mitochondria Meditation.. 52
- Lymphatic Breathing 54
- The Core Supercharger.. 55
- Base Core Supercharger 56
- Empowering the Brainstem 57
- Conehead Meditation 58
- Crown Chakra Meditation 59
- Opening the Base Chakra 59
- The Pot of Gold 60
- The Cosmic Womb 60
- Cerebral Uroboros Meditation 61
- Uni-Phi/Uni-Verse Meditation 62
- The Emancipator 64

CHAPTER 5: FACILITATING THE INNER MARRIAGE...................... 65
- Hemispheric Integration 65
- Upright Walking... 65
- New Thought Walk.. 67
- Noble Posture 67
- Breathing 67
- Core Breathing.. 68
- Fish Breathing... 68
- Bellows Walking... 69
- WHO is Walking?... 69
- Sniff Breathing Walk.. 69
- Serotonin, Grounding and Oxygen 69
- Negative Ion Air... 70
- Maintaining Presence 70
- Turning the Head to the Left 70
- Corebuilding 70
- Repatterning 71
- Click and Drag.. 71

- Cosmic Jellyfish 71
- ORMUS, Mood, Water and Light 71
- Turning Off and Tuning In 71
- The Quantum Bath 72
- The Piss Bath 72
- Emotional Self Regulation 73
- Executive Parenting 73
- Riding Solar Storms 73

CHAPTER 6: NECK AND THROAT 75
- The Primal Scream 75
- Liberating Your Authentic Voice 75
- Hyper-extending the Throat 76
- Opening The Throat 76
- Releasing the Jaw 77
- Get Loud! 78

CHAPTER 7: HEALING THE SPINE 79
- Spinal Opening 79
- Spinal Rebirthing 79
- The Spinal Shower 80
- Hanging 81
- Swan Pose 81
- Solar Sphinx Pose 81
- The Spinal Yoga Roller 82

CHAPTER 8: HEALING THE HEART 83
- Holographic Heart-Field 85
- Whole Brain Consciousness 85
- HeartMath Attitudinal Breathing 86
- Uncaging the Heart 86
- Healing the Heart Hole 86
- Tension Off The Heart 86
- Heart Wings Meditation 87
- Heart Butterfly Meditation 88
- Growing Spiritual Wings 88
- The Heartfield Effect 89
- Arm Shaking Release 89
- Heart Dysautonomia 90
- High Blood Pressure 90

CHAPTER 9: GROUNDING 91
- Touch Ground 94
- Rooting into the Earth 96
- Feeding the Roots 97
- Active Grounding 97
- Personal Grounding Devises 98

- Isometric Stretches 99
- War Haka 100
- Hamstring Stretch 100
- Acumassage Running 101
- The Ass Push Up 101
- Animal Yoga 102
- Kunlun 102
- Kundalini !Kung Dance 103
- Wetter Water 104

CHAPTER 10: REGENERATION EXERCISES 105
- Gratitude 105
- Blue-Sky Club 105
- Freedom Meditation 105
- Substantiation Meditation 106
- Overcoming Inertia To Change 106
- Inner Cosmic Tree 106
- Working with Excalibur, the Silver Cord 106
- Visionary Tune Up 107
- Liver Opening 107
- Solar Rub 107
- Source Charging 107
- Chopping Wood 107
- Embrace the Serpent 108
- Fullness Principles 108
- Unconditional Happiness 108
- Overcoming Addiction to Not Yet and Not Enough 109
- The Sovereign Ground of Being 109
- Divine Play 109

CHAPTER 11: SOCIAL META-ADAPTATION 110
The Clash of Levels 113
- The Crime of Self-negation 114
SOCIAL INNER ARTS PRACTICES 115
- Releasing/Forgiving 115
- Releasing Walk 115
- Attraction Meditation 116
- Serpent Kissing Lovers 117
- Virtual Reunion 117
- King and Queen Pose 118
- The Royal Helm 118
- Positive Projection Practice (PPP) 118
- Substantiating The Holographic Self 119
- Building Left-Brain Efficacy 119
- Sims of Social Success 119
- Pleasure of Devilry 120
- Dealing With Subversive Humor 120

- Turning Shit into Roses 120
- Remaining Conscious 121
- Stance of Social Immunity 121
- Confrontation and Disclosure 122
- Gelassenheit 122
- Compassionate Prayer 123
- Right Livelihood 123
- Truly Serving Others 124
- The Gift of Grace 124
- Self-Hatred, The Principle Poison 125
- Encouraging Others to Find Their Own Way 125
- Self-Care For Social Stress 126
- Agency Willpower Herbs 129

CHAPTER 12: WAKING UP AND SHOWING UP 130
- Methods of Increasing Mental Clarity 133
- How to Spark off Kundalini 134
- Adaptation 135
- Dealing with Acute Kundalini Syndrome 135
- Maintain a Healthy Nervous System 137
- Calm Formula 137
- Nerve Sheaths 138
- Chelation of Heavy Metals and Radionuclides 138
- Radiation Protection 139

END NOTE - ACCENT OF THE INNER MAN 140
THE DIVIDED BRAIN & HINDBRAIN SOCIETY 145
THE TRANSPERSONAL SELF 146
APPENDIX-A: VISIONARY & DREAM WORK 147
APPENDIX-B: SECRETS OF DAILY BLISS 152
APPENDIX-C: TENETS OF DIVINE PLAY 156
RESOURCES 161
BIBLIOGRAPHY 163
ADVANCED MEDIA 164

THE SPHINX

The Sphinx: Tefnut was an ancient Egyptian goddess of moisture, but was strongly associated with both the moon and the sun. The symbol of the Sphinx represents the beginnings of self-reflexive reasoning. Ever since man and woman became self reflective they have wondered about the mystery of life: "Where did it come from and why is it here?"

The Sphinx represents 'all life' and so with equanimity she finds her way through time not caring what form she takes. The Sphinx rises from the unconscious waters of the Uroboros. The Sphinx is a symbol of infinity, or life's attempt to span the ages. Her eternal-primordial wisdom allows her to survive destruction only to rise up phoenix-like from the ashes of unconscious destruction.

The Riddle of the Sphinx, the Rising of the Phoenix, and the search for the Holy Grail and the Elixir of Life are all one and the same. That which allows life to evolve through time and space is the plain and simple truth that "Life comes from Life." This secret of eternal regeneration has been passed on in the mythic symbol of the Sphinx for perhaps 50,000 years.

The Sphinx is a timeless archetypal form representing the nobility, divinity and glory of the life-force itself. At any time the Sphinx will arise as a deeply felt sensation whenever the life-force seeks to break through and enlighten unconscious suffering on the "ways of life." By listening to the source of all life we grow to realize that we do indeed live in a benevolent Universe. Her message is so deep and haunting, she speaks from our very core, yet her whisper shouts through our every pore.

ACKNOWLEDGEMENTS

Thanks to all the people who treated me horribly. It is because of you the Inner Arts were born. Thanks to all the people who treated me beautifully. It is because of you that I had the strength to write this book. And thanks to all the people who get something out of this book and carry on the Inner Arts in their own unique way.

THE INNER ARTS

EXERCISES FOR KUNDALINI INTEGRATION, AWAKENING AND SOVEREIGNTY

INTRODUCTION

Respecting the sovereignty of others arises automatically as we respect our own personal sovereignty.

There comes a time when it becomes impossible to go on as you used to. When you have to step back and stop wasting time on the insignificant. Bonding to the inner cosmos of the interior Self is the new frontier and the most immediate necessity to the fulfillment of the actual needs of Being. The Source Intelligence that fosters all life is the energetic electromagnetic life-force that is intrinsic to our ability to achieve and sustain conscious evolution into the new paradigm. The greater the energy supply of Source Intelligence we are able to integrate and incarnate into embodied presence the more enlightened and sovereign we become. The ultimate technology is an inside job, undertaken by the sovereign human being plugging into the wheel works of Nature.

That all riches lie within becomes apparent when we start doing the Inner Arts in nature—mating our energy with the earth's ions, the sun's photons, with the moon, the water, plants, wind, seasons and the elements. This book contains inner psychotropic exercises for the energetic coupling of body, mind, soul and cosmos, and thereby amplifying our conscious participation in Source Intelligence. The Inner Arts are neuroemotional kinesthetic, meditative techniques specifically for building connection to the core sovereign Self. These sovereignty Inner Arts practices will help us create new neural pathways, and greater skills for thriving in this time of cultural reconstruction.

The Inner Arts practices are for generating harmonious biology, peaceful emotions and blissful frequencies. This harmonious shift to cosmic sympathetic resonance then translates into beneficent life experience and behavioral change. By incorporating sovereignty practice into our daily life we increase communication on all scales from subatomic through to galactic, whereby we transform our instrument, and so transform our lives. The Inner Arts exercises are a playful experiential exploration of intimate communication with our the cells of the body in the ecstatic Vortexijah of the Solar Heart. Through harmonious cosmic connection there is a direct awareness, a grokking, and a knowing, without the need to know, which is the simple relaxed recognition of "what is." If we remain locked in the head, without building subtle felt-sense throughout the body, our reality is fractured in the chaotic, conflicted maelstrom of the compartmentalized self.

Felt-perception can travel deeper and deeper into the body until it touches and awakens a parts of our organism previously dormant. Breaking through one energy valence to another often releases anger and frustration as we become conscious of how we are repressing and numbing ourselves. With increased breath, movement and felt-perception we touch our self-betrayal and so there is often guilt and grief associated with throwing off our armor. Aerobics, strength training, stretching, martial arts and bodywork will help us get through our inertial resistance to dearmoring, to keep the opening process moving along indefinitely. Sovereign self-betrayal produces inevitable biological guilt and yet in false-power societies we are trained to be loyal to external authorities rather than our inner connection to Source. Thus shame and intimidation is the goo that holds the structure of Borg power-pyramid in place by exploiting our fundamental sense of guilt from self-betrayal.

Shame and exclusion tap into our infantile fear of abandonment—and this break in the social bonding mechanism is the underlying cause of the fragmentation of the entire human cosmos. Shaming as a method of social control is always medieval as it is arises from the morally deficient Hindbrain. Power-driven culture comprises of mythic fabrications and untruths that reject the irrevocable fact of the personal sovereignty or divinity of each individual. Biological shame, disappointment and the consequent self-abandonment and self-abnegation inherent in the Borg state is held in the holding patterns of our physical matrix. It is this that drives the socioeconomy of fear, scarcity and addiction. Shame short-circuits deservability, self-worth, claiming our space and the sense of the "right to life" necessary for the sovereign connection to source.

Shame gets caught in the rhomboids between the scapulas. It occurs in association with guilt, which is held in the contraction around the adrenal glands and the diaphragm, essentially cutting us off from any possibility of Flow or the sovereign connection to source. Flow is de-repression—the opposite of somatic shame…it is pulling out all the stops, while depression is self-oppression, the opposite of Flow. Along with the diaphragm and the Iliopsoas muscle, opening up the rhomboids to free the spiritual wings of the heart is essential to spiritual life. Until our spiritual wings are flight worthy, we remain a prisoner of the immoral control mechanisms of Borg psychosis that violates the sovereign divinity of others via "medieval shaming" for malevolent control.

Emotions, sensations, feelings and qualia aren't irrational, they have their own inevitable logic—we just have to bring them into the light of day, understand them, raise them up, refine them and beatify them. Emotions, sensations, feelings and qualia reveal to us what is Real about our subjective experience. The only freedom is the Real. When we are real we can change the instrument of our sensing and sentience such that our emotions, sensations, feelings and qualia toward being life enhancing and uplifting. Thus if we change our felt-sensing of reality we change our reality. Conversely we can intend, go through the motions, appear functional and have positive cognitive thoughts, but if we have not positively engaged our sensual and emotional bodymind our life is still flat, false, representative, abstract and lacks meaning.

Because presovereign Borg society is outer-focused, emotionally repressed and resistant to original thought—the Inner Man is left undeveloped. Since the neural wiring for inner communication is sparse the "music" of consciousness creation fails to pick up enough alchemical momentum to raise the individual beyond the first three chakras so to speak. Hence the overwhelming preponderance of 5-Sense Flatland materialism and rote religiosity, rather than mystic bliss and unique, sovereign creativity.

How about owning one's self and refusing to be a victim of contrived cultural conditions that undermine our potential for evolved humanity? When you sing your own unique song you emit your own frequency rather than being a sponge for the frequencies of other people's reality. To avoid creating reality that paradoxical or contrary to our desires, we must first vibrate in the frequency of attainment or success around the object of desire. When we are not our aligned with our true Self we are a composite being with diffuse ambiguous intent our energy signature is thus confused and diffused. But when we align with our true nature, we overcome the anxiety of separation and the Universal Will and our personal will become one. Thus happenstance becomes happystance.

We transcend the unending onslaught of ignorance and power-abuse of the Borg by strengthening and exercising the higher brain wiring, and raising our cellular energy. We gain immunity from the inertial gravity of the Borg once we can plug ourselves back into full sensory awareness of the energetic ground of the cosmos…ie: Presence. Borg consciousness is composed of habits of memory, imagination and anticipation – largely geared towards sense gratification and escaping the constant inner conflict and anxiety. While the labile, sovereign Presence awareness is tuned into and autopoetically follows the Muse arising from the Beyond.

Grokking and gnosis is the difference between learning with the brain, and learning with the Total HUman. This is where Psi, apotheosis and eureka come in during kundalini awakening — as "bliss producing insights" alchemically transform the bodymind. Eurekas and the kundalini inner conjunction are the two most intense experiences that light up the pleasure centers. Psi goes up at night when the earth shields us from the sun and also during solar quiet periods, this is symbolic of the Inner Janus, or interiorization. Apparently you can increase Psi thru doing the white powder of gold initiation. But then several months of fasting will do the same.

Increasing your cell voltage and removing the insulating layers of plaque, toxins, excess fat and pathogens will increase Psi — raising the frequency on your dial up towards more ethereal levels of cosmic consciousness — or perfect communication with the Unified Field of consciousness. Running or aerobic exercise is necessary for both increasing metabolic rate and detoxification, so movement is necessary for entering into mystic-visionary level reality. So long as there is no vision, there can be no real change. Aerobic exercise is both excellent for extracting our being from the toxic, corrosive influence of the Borg and for amplifying the all aspects of creativity, both for inception, conception, execution and expression. I would say that the combination of remineralization, use of exotic matter (ORMUS), fasting and heart pumping exercise are essential to pick up spiritual speed enough to break away from the gravity of the Borg. Perhaps if the human primate body is not exposed to movement - falling, flying, jumping, climbing, swinging and hanging - then we live life with the brakes on.

That which is not lived out physically becomes mental, emotional and spiritual constipation. The pattern of our life reflects the level of subtle dexterity and the strength of our physical form. However we cannot be healed from the solely physical perspective, for becoming whole requires an integrated multi-dimensional approach that encompasses everything from soil to soul. Focus on removing social-PTSD (psychosexual shaming, disgust, repulsion, trauma) from the bodymind is vitally important at this point in our social evolution and this requires peaceful society. Faith in HUmanity and the gradual development of social forms and institutions increases the sovereign potential of individuals and so we really need a nova of Eros, embodied cognition and social response-ability to overthrow the dark night of rising material fascism. The origin of distress, disease and dysfunction lies in the disturbance of this integrated functioning of the higher intelligence of the body.

The Inner Arts are about improving the capacity to move through the world in an empowered and creative way and to expand the depth of play in our life. In order to attain the sustenance of divine integrity we must have transcended narcissism of Borg psychosis and truly be plugged into the cosmogenetic frequency of love and our own unique genius. To become fully HUman we must establish equanimity in dealing with shadow and embracing the light—thus gaining freedom from the machinations of the Borg, by not resonating with its fallen nature. The Given world is the default program of the Borg. We free ourselves from the Borg by unleashing the vital *Psi* powers of the imagination. It is after all dysfunctional to subconsciously comply with dysfunction. Through dearmoring and holistic development we seek to remove the subconscious repression born of the presovereign's fear of freedom, and in this way we reduce our own suffering, the suffering of others and the suffering of all life.

I am looking for an international ecommerice entrepreneurial genius to license a revolutionary product that will help humanity evolve into a peace-loving species. Please email me if anyone is interested in the ultimate fun and VERY lucrative international business that will supply the investment capital for launching Civilization Next!
jananz@hotmail.com

CHAPTER 1
THE INNER ARTS

SOVEREIGNTY PRACTICES FOR THE INNER COSMONAUT

"Once the Inner Arts goes mainstream, the human species will collectively get more bio-energy and wisdom, hence less opportunity for oppression, war and poverty...it's a big dream!" Debbie M.

The "Inner Arts" are tools for unblocking body armor—for even if we up our energy levels, unless we work directly on dearmoring then all we have is increased metabolic energy inside a fossilized, rigid and neurotic body. Thus we have to work on both the mitochondria energy production, detoxification, remineralization and nutrient density, aerobics, increasing inner communication and an ever-increasing exploration of the "edge" of the body-cage. Basically to penetrate through the "noise" you hold a focused position in the Inner Arts exercise until the higher frequency is imprinted and you feel an AHA!

The reason why the Inner Arts are done outside is that our current architecture not life enhancing (biogenic). Only nature heals, and provides the energy needed to change, grow and raise our frequency. Only nature provides the correct energies and combinations of frequencies needed to facilitate self-communication within the Inner Man and thus conduct full spectrum consciousness. Human degeneration and trauma is mostly instigated and propagated inside man-made structures and man-made cities—that is, electromagnetic structures which are currently not conducive for maximal consciousness or physical, mental and spiritual health. Thus we cage ourselves within physical, mental, social and cultural constructs that prevent the emergence of the full HUman. We then have to spend the majority of our efforts compensating for the damage done by these unnatural aberrations. In order to rectify the ever-increasing distress of human decline, we first have to work on reHUmanizing according to cosmic design and then set about creating a culture that supports the genuine spiritual evolution of humanity and the exuberant health of the planet.

The more the Inner Arts are practiced the less socio-economic, status and relationship stress pulls us out of coherent alignment and the more resilient we are to addictions that disrupt our biology and make it impossible to gain a strong, focused presence in the body. When our biochemistry is stable and coherent creating a grand synthesis of body-mind-soul, holding our own and steering our own course becomes automatic. With substantiation, "timing and synchronicity" reach magical-daemonic proportions and we really start to live the mystery of the sovereign life.

The Inner Arts and other spiritual practices boost the immune system, potentiate the endocrine system, support neurogenesis and neuroplasticity and epigenetically turn on genes for positive emotional states. Running, novel environments, adventure and antidepressants can ramp up neurogenesis of the hippocampus, while stress, social isolation, sleep deprivation and aging can shut it down. By exorcising the duplicit, conflicted, neurotic tyrant out of our bodymind with the Inner Arts, we build up the compassionate, embracing, inclusive executive capacity and the push-pull of inner divisiveness is dissolved.

Once we have conquered hyper-reactivity, inner conflict, inferiority complex, weakness and helplessness we begin to operate in an integrated fashion as our own Guru and lover—our own "Sovereign." This synthesis of sympathetic resonance is geometrically progressive, bringing greater depth, meaning, interest, purpose and agency to our lives. That is we become truly enchanted beings by dearmoring and exorcising our demons. Through active dearmoring we learn that our pain-body and our shadow, negativity or lower self is not something to fear, but when transmuted becomes a doorway to spiritual awakening. Thus through the journey of creative emergence, our deepest wounds become our greatest gifts and greatest teachers.

Raising our energy frequency beyond reactive mind towards creative imagination constitutes the beginning of the spiritual life.

INNERDIMENSIONAL JOURNEYING

THE KINESTHETIC INNERCEPTIVE SENSES

The Inner Arts arose out of my efforts to maintain my wholeness and integrity in a world that seems to want to tear me apart and use me for its own questionable purposes. The discovery of sovereignty Inner Arts involved getting triggered by Hindbrain behaviors so that an Inner Art would emerge from within to ease my suffering. Most of the Inner Arts self-generate from bumping up against the sadomasochistic walls of the Borg in some way. Thus the Inner Arts are a form "internal yoga" practice for integrating kundalini energy and awaken sovereignty (Self-realization). Through the unblocking and harmonizing our energy we can change the fundamental inertial patterns holding us back from realizing our vast potential. The first stage is building the neurology for the integration of kundalini energy, then and there is a need to build the nervous system for self-will and communication with the higher mind. The Inner Arts for the third phase, of building the visionary-neurology, have not be included in this book as they have not yet arisen out of the ether.

These sovereignty practices are not to be limited to being used merely as a band-aid, but can be adopted as a foundation for achieving meta-adaptation… that is to create a life of our choosing that serves the higher good. It requires mindful motivation to stick with the program and assimilate spirituality into every day life, rather than falling into regressive maladaptive fear modes. The effectiveness of these meditations and practices is reduced if we have eaten too much cooked food or otherwise reduced consciousness or clogged energy flow — then the meditation can still be done but it has little effect. Practice when devitalized or occluded is like spinning our wheels and going nowhere. We get out of it what we put into it. Each session is different depending on one's diet, fitness, ability to concentrate, and harmonic coherency at the time.

PHI TRANSFIGURATION

Transfiguration or transmutation means to change into a different shape or form, and kundalini fire rebirths and shapeshifts us more completely than anything else. The building of a sovereign body with kundalini is rather like muscle building. It is a balancing act of vitalizing, integrating, grounding, detoxification and bodywork. The aim of spiritual practice, discipline and lifestyle is not to generate specific phenomena, but to "allow" whatever phenomena to arise according to its own cosmic timing or Kairos (God's time). For example progressive fasting gets rid of the majority of the blockage to spiritual frequencies and peak experiences.

As our cell voltage rises we see light phenomena through the synesthesia of body and the clairvoyant nature of the brain to generate visions. The great illuminated geniuses like Tesla and Walter Russell for sure had this ability of internally seeing psychic imagery directly from the Void so to speak. Transcendental vision is the highest frequency produced in the brain via the Spirit Molecule DMT.

"When we are slaves of the reactive mind we are not really "human" we are just humanoid." Urgyen Sangharakshita

The Borg conditioned brain spends enormous effort repressing the chemical cascade for spiritual consciousness. The extent of our pain-body is equivalent to the cruelty and ignorance in the methods and mechanisms that we use to avoid the realization of who we really ARE. The key to success with the Inner Arts is knowing that they are for cultivating full sensorial intelligence. The term "Phi-synesthesia" hints at the multidimensional, multi-perspectival nature of transcendental consciousness, which is a full spectrum sensory and metasensory apperception. Apperception *(from the Latin, ad-: "to, toward" and percipere: "to perceive, gain, secure, learn, or feel")* means to Grok or conscious perception with full awareness that engenders understanding of newly observed qualities of an object or amplification of subjective experience. Thus Grokking is perceiving or receiving through beginner's mind. The word Grok is related to an ancient meaning of the word "understand" which means to "stand under" another's experience and worldview, like a mystic or artist whom enters into another's direct field of awareness.

Stepping into our power we breed confidence — (fidelity and faith). Owning our own authority in life or "Brain brightness" is measured and experienced in **Clarity** (coherence), **Energy** (mV), **Light** (Lux), **Focus** (depth of field), and **Happiness** (openness), **Information** (connection) and **Flexibility** (plasticity). When shifting from a life resonating in the Borg frequencies to a sovereign life you need to watch your brain brightness and your breathing, if either of those are interfered with then some form of inquiry, direction change, skill acquisition or social turn-about is needed. Then as you feel the stress, agitation or sleepiness ask yourself what needs to occur in your inner and outer environment to bring you back into harmony, Presence, joy, peace and aliveness.

We get the light flowing by removing the blocks and amp energy production, Nature-synesthesia and cosmic-connection. Then we no longer personify Sisyphus - endlessly trying to push our massive rock of dysfunction up hill. Use Phi magically and we fly up the hill without the rock of self-oppression. *The Borg IS sadomasochism personified, ie: pleasure from negative or life harming means.* It is all about win/lose, top/bottom, and "taking" in order to "use." If we can fully unpack the mechanism of sadomasochism we can free ourselves from it, and so set free Eros from the death grip of Thanatos. What the Hindbrain cannot conceive in its limited scope is that when we "use" we are "used," and so we lose, for we expend energy in "taking." We are used by that which we attempt to use because we are attached to that which we are taking and from whom we are taking it.

Whereas if we are creative we "gain" energy in creating, and then we have more to "share," and giving gives us energy. We begin to break free of the mechanism of sadomasochism once we stop abusing ourselves and allowing ourselves to "used and taken" from by sadistic predators and parasites. It is our tendency to devalue ourselves and treat ourselves as a slave and victim that keeps us fate bound within the power pyramid paradigm, without the energy, creativity or resources to break free. The sovereignty of the individual — indeed the divinity of the individual is the foundation stone of all civilization. If the culture undermines the sovereignty and full potential of the individual, then it is not civilized. People should not have to fight to be themselves, and fight to survive for meager crumbs in a bankrupt system.

Our brains and therefore our lives are crafted by the culture we live in. If we apply ourselves to rebuilding our brain through Inner Arts, meditation, nutrition, and changes in our social and ecological environment we can alter the systemic activation of different areas of the brain that correlate to not this "existing culture," but to an enlightened or mystic culture, or sacred civilization. The death culture is a bad habit that we can overcome with compassionate intention, sensitive intuition, faithful insight and ecstatic vision. Transcending our own personal or collective shadow gives us the hope and discipline to act for the furtherance of life.

Ego is Hindbrain dominance, which is generated from the developmental arrest of living in a power addicted/disempowered civilization. Infantilism is compliance to mediocrity, whereas the sovereign individual IS God. The Inner Arts, prayer and meditation helps us cohere or resonate with the Void, Infinity, and commune with the Universal Creatrix or God within. Funny how we have to stop, get quiet and go within in order to touch non-locality, expansiveness and nobility.

The inner universe is more vast and profound than we could ever imagine, thus we need Inner Arts to explore this limitless territory.

CHAPTER 2

FOUNDATION INNER SKILLS

• STOPPING

We have to stop being who we were, to be who we ARE. I think we have to be schizophrenic (liable) to navigate the collective psychosis of the age, but unless we have disembedded from Hindbrain-dominant state then we are still caught up in the psychotic cultural matrix. As a "follower" we still believe the fleeting figments on Plato's cave wall are real, and so we waste our lives shadow fighting with phantoms that are irrelevant to who we really are. We disembed from Hindbrain dominance by yogic control over the parasympathetic/sympathetic sides of our nervous system. In this sense we start the spiritual life by first stopping the entropic waste of energy from runaway automatic responses to stimuli. The presovereign Borg lacks the executive perspective to STOP reacting and rebounding around in automatic Hindbrain mode. Hindbrain is another term for the fragmented, incoherent or partial consciousness that is caught up in and embedded in the Matrix and asleep to its Givens.

To marry the hemispheres, connect the Triune Brain and get into the self-dominion of the Prefrontal Lobes you have to first clear out the brain stem, and root the head-brain into the solar plexus or enteric-brain, as well as bringing the head into resonance with the Heart. To clear the brain stem you can use the Core Supercharger, and to establish the central nervous system roots you can use the Heart-Tree Meditation.

Besides the Primal Release Pose there are many things you can do to expand the diaphragms capacity and release its tension. Punching, pushing against a wall, stretching with a broom handle, running, huffing, running up stairs, bending your back over a couch arm and breathing hard into the diaphragm. These along with the master integrators—the Blue Spot Meditation and the Mitochondrial Meditation represent the four pillars of sovereignty practice that begin to grow the neurology for the Inner Man. You cannot be anything but a Hindbrain creature if you don't first establish the neuro-emotional framework or the intranet for sovereign consciousness.

• MAKE LIKE A ROCK

A good stopping exercise is to Make Like a Rock. Lie as nude as possible in the sun on slightly damp grass. Start on your back first, simply letting go and feeling the electrons from the earth entering your body, and the sun heating your belly. When you turn over on your stomach feel into the earth and feel the sun healing your kidneys. Imagine you are a rock and let the weight of your body drop into the earth, while letting out strong huffing out-breaths.

• INNER SMILE

It is our holding onto dissonant emotions and frequencies that keeps us in the victimized, helpless contracted state, so we are the only one that can release it. Simply choose to do so by loving yourself enough, and stop punishing yourself for the suffering that should not have been yours in the first place. You melt the distressed state by "growing" out of it with love, light and laughter. One of the fastest ways to break out of victim consciousness is to SMILE! It takes a strong soul not to be distracted by the power trauma-drama. A simple smile has the power to alter the course of human history. Notice that if you are not engaged in climbing on top of anyone, nor submitting to someone climbing on top of you, then you are smiling. So the Inner Smile is the bridge to the transcendent future.

A child born into the distressed, presovereign family has an innate ability to be happy and exuberantly smiling. However while we are still a child and passively reacting to our social environment it is virtually impossible to differentiate ourselves from the family "mood" and undercurrents. Through self-observation and practice we can change the base-tone of our emotional state to be "happier" than our family of origin. I have established a somewhat permanent Inner Smile associated with my kundalini awakened heart—by watering it like a flower with nectar through cultivating the Inner Arts. When doing the Inner Arts it is immediately apparent that we experience a wholesale sea change in consciousness and well-being through doing the Inner Smile. Once we have a well attended heart-field, we have greater readiness in extending our heart nectar and smile to others. It is all about connection with Source.

A smile creates friendly connection in which competency and efficacy are naturally present within the "Go" and the "Yes" inherent in goodwill. The incredible transformative power of a smile can dramatically change social zeitgeist towards happiness because the endorphins produced through a smile makes us feel and look better and positive-forward thinking eradicates the conflict, distress and confusion of "occupying" the reptilian and limbic brains. With a genuine smile the whole-brain mode via the heart-prefrontal lobe connection is established, which is essential to Source fed relationships… thereby supporting health, immunity and humanization itself.

The Inner Smile is the bridge between the reptilian brainstem, limbic-emotional and neocortex-human brains. It also roots the brain into the solar plexus and allows the brain to fall into sync with the primary resonator of the Heart-field. It also balances the hemispheres so that both analytic and intuitive faculties are available. There is no wholebrain consciousness or sovereignty without the Inner Smile. With reconnection practice and mindfulness we can maintain a permanent Inner Smile, however we must also upgrade our daily social environment so that it is not toxic to our higher well-being. Otherwise our Inner Smile will become false and our life like poor Sisyphus, fruitlessly trying to push his stone uphill again and again against overwhelming resistance.

THE THREE KINGS

The Three Kings are incorporated into all Inner Arts practices as a means of "getting inside the body" to regulate and transform. The Three Kings are essential to all Inner Arts to turn on the vagal nerve and activate the Parasympathetic Nervous System or "off switch" in order to do "inner work." The Three Kings involve dropping the muscles at the back of the Tongue, doing a Throaty Breath and an Inner Smile. Dropping the tongue into the belly and breathing is the fastest and surest way of breaking through the contraction and anxiety that constitute surface living. It also automatically reduces hyper-activation of the nervous system in people in our proximity. The parasympathetic mode promotes rest, recovery, healing, growing and visioneering, and can be used to facilitate the art of daily life.

Dropping the muscles at the root of the tongue electrically connects us into the ground of consciousness within the (8Hz)-serotonin, enteric or stomach brain. This then marries the left and right brain hemispheres, plus the Heart with the prefrontal lobes and ultimately the body with the earth and planetary Schumann resonance (8Hz). The Inner Smile creates the endorphins needed to the relaxation of the HPA-axis overdrive and put us in a "growth" state. Raising the vibration beyond the swamp of delusion is about eliminating interference patterns and building coherency.

Once you have sufficient charge, conductivity, coherency and conjugation through eliminating everything that which blocks the light, then the Grace of Spirit is able to descend (incarnate), kundalini sparks up and burns off the rest of the blockage and noise. At which point we are progressively free from the gravity, friction and inertia of the Borg because we have established the ways, means and conditions for maintaining cosmic reconnection. Through fracturing, dissociation and discombobulation the Borg has fallen out of cosmic communion, thus is the Borg is alienated from body, soul and cosmos.

Drop the back of tongue, put on an inner smile and do a throaty breath and the brain shifts into sympathetic/parasympathetic balance or "dual hemisphere mode." You will notice a direct connection to the solar plexus brain and bliss effervescing from the heart through the jaw and into the brain. The eyes soften and radiate with light, essence and pleasure. This simple method of generating whole-brain consciousness can be used throughout the day and night to promote a relaxed, open, optimistic and receptive state with which to engage all life. Bring attention to relaxing your forehead and temples, releasing your inner ears, letting go of your jaw and bringing a steady, soft focus to your eyes.

The Three Kings are the portal to the wholebrain state! Through conscious entry into the inner-kinesthetic sense, then you can go on from there to root the brain into the solar plexus, integrate the root chakra and sex organs into the wholebody sense, ground the feet into the earth, elongate and repolarize the spine, clear the brainstem, plasma charge the brain core, initiate the prefrontals, bathe the bodymind in the heart-field, open the crown to the cosmos, drop social anxiety for all mortals, cleanse and oxygenate the blood and feel fully at home wherever you are.

• DROPPING THE TONGUE (OFF SWITCH)

To come out of fight/flight and into the parasympathetic off switch you drop your tongue into your belly. That is, loosen the muscles at the root of the tongue. This gives the sensation of an immediate connection with the stomach. Focus "peace" into the brainstem — while doing the Inner Smile (for endorphins) — and warm throaty breaths into the solar plexus. Dropping the muscles at the back of the tongue, so that the jaw tension is unleashed is a requisite component of most of the Inner Arts Practices. It is an effective means of immediately turning off sympathetic hyperdrive and dropping monkey mind.

You should notice your stomach gurgling within minutes as the digestive system is activated by the parasympathetic. Since the Borg is glued together through dissociated Beta-wave and Left-brain busyness we fail to get the hyper-relaxation necessary to drop fully into our subterranean layers and come into our full, vibrant Self. If you do the tongue drop, inner smile and throaty breath throughout the day, you will eventually come out of hyper-sympathetic overdrive.

Dropping the tongue into the belly and breathing is the fastest and surest way of breaking through the contraction, dissonance and anxiety that constitute disassociated surface living. It also automatically reduces hyper-activation of the nervous system in people in our proximity. The parasympathetic mode promotes rest, recovery, healing, growing and visioneering.

Dropping the muscles at the root of the tongue electrically connects us into the ground of consciousness within the (8 Hz)-serotonin, enteric or stomach brain — this then marries the left and right brain hemispheres, plus the Heart with the prefrontal lobes and ultimately the body with the earth and planetary Schumann resonance (8 Hz). The Inner Smile creates the endorphins needed to the relaxation of the HPA-axis overdrive and put us in a "growth" state.

• PLUGGING INTO THE SOVEREIGN STATE

Consciousness means nothing if it is not applied. A profound sense of peaceful Presence is experienced when we enter into the deep stillness of our inner being. Dropping the attitude of attachment, aversion and achievement and acquisition. The practice of **The Three Kings**—(tongue drop, inner smile and throaty breath) permits increased oxygen uptake necessary for wholebrain, wholebody consciousness. Basically you drop the muscles at the back of the tongue to release the jaw, this turns on the Vagal Nerve (parasympathetic)... allowing you to do a Throaty Breath with the larynx and trachea open and relaxed. The Inner Smile puts you in Alpha Frequency...the gateway to wholebrain-body inner connectivity. Thus Three Kings allows us to enter our inner domain in order to Know Thyself and engage in inner transformation. We become invincible by practicing The Three Kings and radiant-feeling into the earth and the cosmos. Through progressive relaxation, integration and growth we unify into "Wholebeing," or sovereignty. Deep subatomic relaxation is necessary in generating the coherence and higher field strength to increase the signal-to-noise ratio of consciousness, whereby we plug into the sovereign state.

• GROUNDING = HARMONIZING

Grounding can be done by simply lying on the grass or sand for 1/2 hour a day or taking long barefoot walks in nature. The human foot without footwear is far healthier, is grounded to the electromagnetics of the earth, that alone supports Whole Humanhood. By grounding into the electromagnetics of the earth this improves the immune system, decoagulates the blood, and supports oxygen uptake. If you feel you have sparked up your energy too much with an extreme kundalini event then half an hour swim in the ocean or river will calm down the fire and reintegrate it. If meditation makes you too spacious and ungrounded, then meditate while sitting on the ground in nature, preferably near running water. Use the earth and grass as a free electron, antioxidant source to counter inflammation—even going out first thing in the morning to walk barefoot through the dew, while greeting the rising sun.

• ESTABLISHING THE MIND'S EYE

The mind's eye is used to gain conscious purchase on any area that you focus on and thereby to palpate it and bring it into conscious awareness. By the mind's eye I mean the kinesthetic felt-sense and directional focus of the brain. This feels like a connection between the third eye region and the brainstem. When directing the mind's eye, the closed eyes are pointed in the direction you are focusing on. Thus you can even direct energy (look) out through the back of the eyeballs and down into the brainstem, or in any other direction of focused intent. You can even get the sense that you are flipping your eyeballs over and down into your cerebellum…I used to do this every night as a child to go into bliss while putting myself to sleep.

• TONING

When we hum or Huuu this reverberates through our separate parts, coalescing consciousness. *"Himma"* is an Arab word meaning: meditating, conceiving, imagining, projecting and passionately desiring. Himma raises our being toward focused creative intent through the unifying heart. Our soul's vocation is our creative hymn to divine transportation. Light can be created from sound. We are called Hu-man—for if you tone Huuu, the muscles at the back of the tongue and throat relax and vibrate, relaxing one out of survival mode and into higher "human" sensibilities. The sound reverberates in the head and brain ventricles, speeding the detoxification and feeding of the brain, and adding to greater ionizing/energizing of the cerebrospinal fluid. I cannot stress enough that toning and mantra are the most effective tools we have for integrating energy during an awakening and helping the kundalini to clear through blockages.

Toning and Mantra is the main method of treating consciousness and is helpful for healing all levels of the mind inner and outer. The sound and breath combination help move cerebrospinal fluid which cleanses the brain and spine. Lie in a deep hot bath and hum one tone on the expiration of one breath. You will notice that your tone wavers, perhaps due to the spasticity of the diaphragm. If one continues using this technique regularly perhaps with both higher and lower tones, the diaphragm should strengthen and release its spasticity through the vibration. Joe Alexander says toning works better than any other self-healing tool. I suggest half an hour of toning a day — keep it simple, either *Huuu, Mooo, Om* or *Eeee* will do, or whatever sound you are drawn to.

• SYNCOPATED TONING

One day I found a neat affect when I was sitting down by the river near a little waterfall/rapids, and started to tone Huuu. Then I toned vowel sounds very loud and I noticed that when the tone is directed toward the rapids, the air filled with the sound of the rapids creates an interference pattern with the tone one is emitting and what ends up happening is a staccato vibration in the diaphragm created by the interference pattern of the merging sounds. In this way the effect of toning on the body is greatly amplified when the tone is directed at the noise of the falling water.

When each tone finds Atonement with the river sound the staccato effect is "felt" and heard. If the tone is slightly "off" in relationship to the river the syncopation effect doesn't occur. However the sensitive body-voice naturally tunes to the correct tone — nature the great tuning fork. The syncopated toning I found July 2002 when in extreme horniness with the kundalini — I went down to the river to try and get some relief and found that staccato effect. I was so blown away, I thought I had discovered a new law of the physical universe, of course this distracted me from my oppressive sex energy. Once the diaphragm learns how to do this you can retain the staccato ability even without using a river when the kundalini light is highly active.

• GETTING A GRIP ON THE BRAINSTEM

The brainstem is one of the hardest regions of the body to get a grip on because unless we are cultivating consciousness our "mind" tends to move away from the brainstem as a means to avoid the felt responses of emotion. Thus in this contracted society we are often cut off at the neck and operating with an unconscious body, a barely conscious mind and suppressed feeling and Psi. The brainstem is at the bottom of the *kinesthetic innerceptive sense* of the mind's eye and you can enter it with conscious intent by turning the eye socket muscles back and down into the brainstem. You need to do continuous breath to maintain your grip and it may help to press a hand lightly into this area in order to focus attention.

Whenever fear or conflict arises focus the mind's eye on the brainstem while doing attitudinal heart breathing for peace. This turns off recriminations-defense mind that is associated with flight-fight chemistry. First breathe peace into the heart on the in-breath, then peace down into the brain stem with the out-breath. Doing peace breathing focused into the solar plexus in the bath is especially transforming especially when Toning is used as well. When there is no conflict within, there is no conflict without. The Inner Smile produces endorphins, thereby creating a receptive, impressionable state for emotional reprogramming.

Doing the Inner Smile with the mind's eye focused on the back of the skull at the foramen magnum dip where the spine enters will unblock and organize the energy of consciousness into a coherent flow. By knowing the pathways for apriori wholeness within and establishing Higher Homeostasis we make the core connection to the larva lamp of vitality and mana within. Once we no longer carelessly spill our own light, we can fill up from the inside to rise to unity consciousness — where we are actually contributing our radiance to the world, rather than merely spewing forth our need.

• OPENING THE MOUTH OF GOD

By opening the apex center at the base of the skull, above the first cervical vertebra we allow the full flow of energy-consciousness whereby the lower may harmoniously ascend and spiritual inspiration, or the "Flute of the Gods," the divine logos or voice of the Muse be heard. This "Mouth of God" region, also known as the Jade Pillow by the Chinese, is part of a "pump" that draws cerebrospinal fluid and chi energy upwards from the roots. While lying on your the back place the tips of your three middle fingers in the dip where the spine meets the cranium and with the other hand press the third eye region to apply more pressure to the dip. Drop the muscles at the back of the tongue and do the Inner Smile. Toning Huuu with the mouth open for more resonance or maintain a throaty breath if not toning. Do a contraction of the pelvic floor (Kegel) with each breath and pull the energy up your spine. Continue on with the opening of "The Mouth of God" by taking the hand that was pressing on the forehead and putting it on the solar plexus.

The opening, un-seizing and cleansing of the cerebellum (movement-motivation) at the back of the brain requires plentiful oxygen and water. The detoxifying and integrating this region, allows a more perfect flow of ecstatic energy into and through the brain, allowing our supreme ruler to nurture our cells throughout the entire hierarchy of our body. We cannot be motivated without an ignited motivation center and this requires the full charge from an open, unkinked, ignited spine. Full Epsom Salt sole can be sprayed on the back of the neck during or after this practice to facilitate the unblocking of energy and removal of toxins.

A round disc of shungite pressed into the spine at the occiput while meditating helps to reduce inflammation and agitation in the brain and spine. Lying on your back and putting a piece of shungite on your Third Eye while meditating greatly amplifies the meditative function and results. A shungite necklace, or shungite flat rounds sewn into the inner side of a choker can be an effective way to normalize emotional distress and normalize the energy in the brainsteam and thyroid. Wear a shungite pendant over the Thymus gland to improve the immune system's intelligence. Put shungite stones or discs over areas of the digestive system that are weak or in discomfort. Holding piece of shungite on the gums near a tooth that is infected or weak will normalize the electromagnetics of the mouth, and reduce brain infection/inflammation.

• NOBLE SEAT

I found that during meditation to direct one's eyeballs and attention back into the brainstem that this profoundly increases steadiness, centeredness and nobility. Brainstem mediation is good for centering, soul recovery, boundary formation and general healing of the entire bodymind. Perhaps it focuses consciousness in the occipital lobes which are the main centers for visual processing, and are serotonin based, contributing to integration and harmony.

• BELLY LOVE

The axel point of the harmony of the spheres is centered in the Hara (lower Tan Tien) in which reverence and equanimity are cultivated as the ground state of being through which the higher self or cosmic being can download into manifest reality. During meditation if one turns the eyeballs directly down into the cheek area the energy flow is directed down into the belly. The belly is then nurtured with energy and a greater connection is achieved between the heart and the belly increasing digestive health and emotional equilibrium and awareness. Using the hands as jumper cables, with one hand on the heart and the other on the belly, will help direct healing love into the area.

• RELAXATION RESPONSE

Meditation is good for the heart—During meditation, the body produces nitric oxide, the chemical used by pharmaceutical companies to lower blood pressure. Prior to receiving any relaxation training in stress management techniques there was no association between oxygen consumption (VO2) slope and nitric oxide. After training, the depth of the elicited relaxation response was associated with increased concentrations of nitric oxide and a significant reduced level of serum fat peroxidation than control group. The relaxation response may be mediated by nitric oxide "opening" of the cardiovascular system helping to explain its clinical effects in stress-related disorders and reducing cardiovascular risk factors.

• DANCE

We come to dance with an imposing idea, yet waiting within there is a dance that awaits to dances us. Those that hold latent psycho-spiritual power are subconsciously terrorized into a straight-jacket of self-suppression by the arrogance and caustic nature of power-over and usury. In the Powerhoe Borg culture the ignore-ance of false power and status poisoning is still almost 100% and so it goes on unabated. It is up to those that hold back their atomic power and make themselves small to fit into the existing prison planet—to set themselves free. We have no idea what that looks like in dance, in speech, in behavior and in social activism—because few ever give themselves permission to truly set themselves free. We have no choice now, we MUST let the dance, dance us WHOLE.

• SUNGAZING

> "Gazing directly into the sun actually improves sight and aids in overcoming disease..." ~ Herbert Shelton.

By using the sun for meditating, the photons dissolve inner conflict, and defrag the brain and so you are left with a clean thinking machine—then this trumped up conflict you are having IS no more. You are under the illusion that your thoughts are reality, when really your computer just needs a good ol' wipe by mother nature. Moonlight and sunlight meditation/gazing spiritually charges and uplifts…providing the fuel for rapid ascension. Sungazing offers improvements in detoxification, health, libido, intelligence, spiritual opening, intuition, creativity and physical energy. It is recommend that you start off with a few minutes a day and increase the duration by a few minutes more each sunny day, building toward sessions 15 minutes or more.

Sunlight increases blood calcium and phosphate, improves of blood oxygen utilization, improves of blood flow properties, and enhanced phagocyte capacity of white blood cells. Sunbathing heals cancer by building up the immune system and increasing oxygen levels in the tissues. It is the damaged molecules from cooked food in combination with sunlight that causes cancer. The sun is needed for vitamin D creation, making sex hormones, mineral assimilation and utilization, building muscle, catalyzing chemical reactions in the body, building strong immune system and bones…and all life processes in the body. Even difficult to remove toxins like lead, cadmium, mercury, liver poisons and neurotoxins were detoxified from 2 – 20 times faster.

In his book *Daylight Robbery: The Importance of Sunlight to Health*, Dr. Damien Downing shares research from Russia that shows that animals exposed to the higher amounts of sunlight were capable of removing toxins out of their body considerably faster than animals reared away from the sun. The Native American tradition believed that if you look at the Sun and go to the heart and appreciate the Sun's contribution to life, and then ask in prayer for a request to be fulfilled or answer to be known.

Sungazing is always done at the hour of sunrise or sunset and seated barefoot, ideally in nature. I've also found that my heartbeat changes when I'm sungazing, always done with a sense of profound connection and gratitude for the sun. *"When you look at the Brightest One, your heart melts in love."* Also I discovered that sungazing is an excellent way to achieve a state of no thought.

The photons from the sun can help soothe and enlighten so that body, mind and soul can enter sympathetic resonance. The sun's rays "defrag," remove imbalances and organize the electromagnetic matrix of living beings. However sungazing/sunbathing or radiation/oxidation in general is damaging to the body if the tissues are made of unstable transfats and your omega-3:omega-6 ratio is off, and you do not have adequate antioxidants from colorful fruits and vegetables in your body reserves.

• MOON GAZING

Basically the moon informs/in-forms on the deepest levels through the energy (passion) on the heart. I haven't found a greater force for insight than the October and November full moons. You can start off by asking a question, but this may be more surface material. Then you might just go with a more nebulous evocation of the sincere, focused devotional heart towards the moon and see if "something" arises. If nothing presents itself don't worry, because it is the "relationship" with the energy of the moon itself, the deep electromagnetic connection and the resulting empathy, passion, glory and awe that matters (literally matters).

• ELIMINATING ENERVATION

Reduce stimulants, cut back on fruit %, increase greens and kelp for minerals, and drink heaps of water. Get plenty of nature and exercise. Preferably one has done ones major cleansing and fasting prior to the onset of kundalini. Avoid energy sapping people, situations, and environments and continually drop the contents of the mind and move onto your highest vision. Paradoxically the chemistry of awakening can lead to a down cycle of anesthesia, apathy, lassitude, lethargy, narcosis, numbness and stupefaction. The torpor can be overcome in the same way it is usually done—jumping in cold rivers, oceans, saunas and cold showers, walking in nature, lying on the ground.

Percussion massage, tapping the head and face, new novel experiences, dancing. B complex vitamins, 6-8g Vitamin C per day with DHLA (dihydrolipoic acid), raw foods, green vegetables and wheatgrass juice. Constant stretching, moving, exercising throughout the day with conscious deep breathing. Drink lots of water, up to 5 quarts a day and pop spirulina tablets throughout the day.. You have to turn your consciousness into the torpor, ask for insight, and invite yourself to be over it. Try Yerba mate tea for work, but don't allow yourself to use substances stimulate yourself out of torpor, for it requires a comprehensive enlivening program that includes super-nutrition, movement, grounding and breathing as its foundation.

• ILEOCECAL VALVE

The upright human pose means that peristalsis has to work against gravity in order to get chyme up to the hepatic flexure. There's a "dead point" in the colon near the ileocecal valve - known as the cecum. This acts like a backwater - and is the top spot in the colon for infections, parasites and stagnant material. Located between the small and large intestine, this valve is usually kept closed so that the food you've eaten stays in your small intestine long enough to be digested and absorbed fully. It also prevents the good microorganisms in your large intestine from getting into your small intestine, where their waste products could easily be absorbed.

When your ileoceal valve is weakened by constipation, poor nutrition and excess food, the yeast and bacteria that live in the large intestine get through the valve and up into your small intestine, where they become "bad bacteria." 90% of Candida establishes itself on the intestinal wall, especially around the ileocecal valve connecting the small and large intestine. A weak ileocecal valve and candida infestation will make the right side of the GI tract by the hip bone sore and bloated.
• Massaging in the morning while still in bed with an electric massage tool is one method of assisting the anatomical distress.
• Morning and evening lie head down on a slant board and massage in circular motions from the ileocecal valve, up the ascending colon on the right side, across the transverse colon and down the descending colon…around the abdomen in a clockwise motion.
• Squat first thing in the morning for 10 minutes while looking at email and Facebook or web news. Squatting realigns the pelvic geometry so that the abdominal muscles are brought more fully into use throughout the day.

- **PM CLEANSER** — Equal parts Psyllium powder, Bentonite Clay, Yucca root powder, Magnesium citrate powder, and Papain or Bromelain enzyme power. Before bed drink 1 tsp of this mix in water, or sparkling water with a little cranberry or prune juice.

MEDITATION AND NEURO-ENHANCEMENT

The brain, and consequently the mind itself, is easily changeable and highly influenced, especially by meditation. On what and how we place our attention affects the growth of our brain, through neuroplastic alterations in the central nervous system, which then automatically shifts our minds and vice versa in a feedback cycle. The directed consciousness effects of "mindfulness" meditation produce a significant improvement in critical cognitive skills such as the ability to sustain attention and vigilance after just four days of training for only 20 minutes each day. Focusing on the flow of breath at the tip of the nose, while letting go of thoughts through attending to the sensations of the breath, trains us to forgo distraction and focus on the task at hand.

Mindfulness Meditation thus improves the brain's neuroplasticity, or ability to adapt to environmental changes and reverses the usual process of aging. Meditation or communion also reduces pain, grows grey matter, increases cortical thickness, enriches brain structures with stronger connections between brain cells, and a higher degree of folding in the cortex, which enhances neural processing. The more folding that occurs the more efficient the brain is at processing information, making decisions, forming memories. The more communication between the older subconscious and newer conscious regions of the brain means there is more "top down" regulation of limbic and autonomic functions. The cortex's executive control plays an integrative role between the limbic, frontal, parietal and temporal lobes, which enhances the subtle abilities of introspection, awareness as well as emotional control and self-regulation.

Without the development of the prefrontal lobes, the person lacks stability, substantialness and focus, and will remain dependent and pupae-like rather than Self-actualized. That is the spiritual power and Presence is diminished without prefrontal development. Prefrontal development occurs when the individual steps out into the world autonomously, without safety nets and crippling dependencies. Without this initiation into mature adult life one's brain is essentially damaged or latent. The prefrontal cortex functions as a conscious awareness (or witness) or reasoning center for impulse control, self-discipline, formulating language, memory, socialization, and the assessment of threat, reward, trust and empathy.

Perhaps it is through the "development" of the brain by meditation that we can gain conscious control or dominion of the powerful drives and impulses that can become pathological when they are unconscious, compulsive and addictive. Thus we see that meditation is one of the most valuable tools a sovereign can use to overcome addiction and compulsion strengthen spiritual muscles.

Self-empowerment is achieved when our meditation practice is centered into the body, calming and bringing it into sympathetic resonance. That which is not out of control can then be bought into concert to support the symphony of the whole. Alterations in brain neurophysiology produce a "transcendent" experience resulting in a simultaneous experience of extreme fulfillment and intense significance (valence)—equating to a profound mystical experience. Stress, the fear response and PTSD increases glutamate release in the hippocampus, while meditation changes the concentration and release of glutamate in the brain from places that promote instability to areas that promote calm.

Meditation's strengthening effects on the brain both reduces subsequent PTSD damage from current trauma, and acts to derepress trauma we may have encountered in the past allowing it to heal. Essentially what this does is to defragment, unseize and youthify the brain, allowing for greater efficiency, spontaneity, increased energy flow and new learning—which translates as increased well-being, happiness and success. *Meditation increases the proficiency in which neurons fall into sync, deepening the sense of self-remembering and ripening the embodiment of the soul.*

• ROOTING THE PREFRONTALS

Maintain a pinch-like hold at the very top of the nose, and very top of the spine, this gives an anchor allowing meditative access to the prefrontal lobes by turning up the eyeballs to the top of the hairline. The neck is held like when a cat lifts her kittens. Pinching the nose and neck simultaneously allows energy to be anchored during the often difficult task of bringing energy into the forehead. Low energy and inflammatory dissonance in the nerves means inefficient mental processes which lowers our Presence, sovereignty and soul-navigation. Sniffing while doing this clears the sinuses.

• CLEARING THE ATTIC

The glymphatic system must be clear and flowing for the feeding of the brain with new blood and energy. This is especially important as it relates to the crown and our connection to the cosmos. The glymphatic system (crown chakra) becomes dull giving us a sense of cosmic separation when we eat late at night, fail to get enough fresh air and exercise or when we endure ongoing psychological abuse from authority figures who have no idea (nor potential for conception) of who and what we are.

One way to open the **glymphatic Mohawk** is to roll the crown of cranium on the ground. Do a crouch by sitting on your legs, similar to both when praying to Mecca and the Rabbit's Pose in yoga. However, the hands are out in front like the Sphinx Pose. Now bend over and carefully roll the top of your head over the carpet, without hyperextending the back of the neck, while sniffing to clear the sinuses.

Make sure you gently roll your Mohawk region from the forehead to the posterior fontanelle region. Hanging from the hips and serpentine movement of the spine around also helps to open the brain's glymphatic highway. Most importantly though, **is to become so ALIVE**, that the social psychosis and competitive, exploitative power wrangling doesn't gravitate in our direction and clog up our cerebral hardware.

Narcissism is simply the material human fallen from the cosmic soul connection. Once opened and released, "connected" and communicating our brain can naturally work to spontaneously create the best of possible lives. Whatever the situation, self-realization gives us the expansive safe space we need to heal and grow. The way to free ourselves from the arrested development of the hive-mind of the Borg is to open up and expand our own higher HUman capacities.

ADVANCED HUMAN CHARACTER TRAITS

Honesty, Fairness, Tolerance, Fortitude, beyond Ego-defensiveness, Joy, Peace, Generosity, Magnanimity, seeks to Further All Life, Faith-Trust, Patience, Universal Compassion and motivated by Kindness, Self-discipline, Chastity, and speaking Truth to Power. Along with these traits are psychic abilities such as Precognition and Visions, Expansive Dream Life, Creative Genius, Telepathy, Reading Minds, Medical Intuition, Ability to Heal, Ubiquitous Desire to Assist All Beings, Fair Witness or Universal Judicial Capacity; plus a Visceral Understanding Of Nature, the Tao and the Fibonacci Nature of Cosmic Design, and invariably inflamed with a Inspired Soul Vocation.

> *"True strength and power and usefulness are born of self-purification, for the lower animal forces are not lost, but are transmuted into intellectual and spiritual energy."* By James Allen, Dignity and Self-Discipline
> www.renegadetribune.com/

The paradigm of destruction that is presently killing the planet is governed by narcissism. Narcissism makes us malleable and vulnerable to the directives of the empire's mind control. Goodness explodes beyond the boundaries of "the control system." Goodness arises from a clear glymphatic system in the brain, that "clears out our attic," and allows for an expanded EMF egg of the body, which connects us to the wider cosmos beyond both the personal and collective sphere. Narcissism, materialism, war-capitalism, empire and all aspects of Borgism are propagated by a **"dirty attic,"** aborting our HUmanity and cutting us off from cosmic design and sacred Destiny.

It is recommended you put a soft plush carpet near your bed, so you can roll your cranium on it before you sleep, and when you first get out of bed in the morning. This is an easy habit to program, and it makes for far deeper sleep and more soul orientation and navigation during your day. Clearing the Attic allows us to disengage from material enslavement and the commodified world, which gives us access to free will, and the discipline to improve spiritually rather than mindlessly following the flock.

Basically I am saying that clogging up your glymphatic system by eating late at night, when coupled with experiencing the stress of social pathology acts to "cut us off from God," unless we undertake lymphatic detox practices. When we run from social toxicity, predators, parasites or power-plays in general we may stagnate our lymphatic system in order to go unconscious so that we numb ourselves out against emotional pain. However by doing so we fail to develop more advanced social adaptive skills and merely prolong "victim energy," which sets us up for further abuse in the future. Clearing the Attic is a simple daily exercise we can do to maintain mindfulness around the need to keep our glymphatic system open and flowing. Sovereignty and self-determination is the only way to arrive at a transcendent destiny.

WHOLEBRAIN GAMMA WAVE

The danger of socioeconomical submission to the power-over dynamic is that it destroys the Wholebrain functioning by which individuals may rise above the subversion of their will by more power-hungry others. If we subordinate our will to that of a dominator, then we fall out of sync with the natural state of cosmic coherence and Truth, Beauty and Goodness…which comes only from the individual's sacred sovereign connection to the cosmos divine.

If the body is a musical instrument for the symphony of consciousness, then when the cell membranes are made rigid by heated fats, and tissues become laden with plagues, growths and pathogens, then proteins and DNA coagulate through acidity and toxicity. The integrity of the cell and self is undermined by morbid accumulations and mutagenesis and the symphony of consciousness falls flat and becomes cacophonous. The harmonious chorus of choruses, is the symphony of the neurons resonating in synchrony to bring about the "awareness" aspect of consciousness through Wholebrain functioning in a neuro-endocrinally complete organism.

Creating the whole HUman involves generating sympathetic resonance right down at the quantum level, on upwards to the regeneration and noospheric regenesis of the planetary consciousness. The concept of the "Harmony of the Spheres" connotes the idea that the whole cosmos, with its circling planets and stars, is in some way a harmonious symphony. Ultimately through the unified field there is no separation, no "I and Thou" in the universe. Genius in all its multitudinous forms is falling into harmonious sync with the music of the spheres. We become cosmic beings and enter cosmic consciousness though attuning ourselves to the rhythm and symphony of the cosmos.

Our self-reflexive intelligence resides in the large area of the cerebral cortex and the amount and number of brain cortical convolutions. Some say that the central organizing executive is somewhere in the frontal lobe of the brain, the part that has most lately developed in evolution. But it is far more likely that what we actually perceive as a unitary, non-fragmentary experience of Self is organized in much the same way as a symphony.

The unitive state of peace and Presence is mediated by a neural network that is well distributed throughout the brain. Focused awareness or meditation trains the prefrontal cortex, to be more mindfully in the present and therefore to spend less time anticipating threats and future negative events. Meditators are less depressed, they anticipate less pain and find pain less unpleasant for they spend less negative energy in resisting it.

Gamma wave or (30 to 90 hertz or cycles per second) rhythms most probably generated by intra-laminar thalamocortical cells characterizes waking and REM sleep. Sensory data, as a general rule doesn't make it to the brain, except through the thalamus. So the thalamus drives or is the prime mover of upper brain levels. The *Locus Ceruleus* of the Pons secretes norepinephrine and is implicated in the arousal aspect of REM or dream sleep. While the serotoninergic Raphe involved in slow brainwave deep sleep may oppose the norepinephrinergic Locus Ceruleus.

Connection or "communication through coherence" is the vibe of "Love." The German neurophysiologist Pascal Fries, states that neuron communication occurs via neuronal synchronization or coherence. Synchronization involves gamma, theta and beta waves, which work together in the brain to produce the various types of human consciousness. Shared electrical oscillation rates, allows for smooth communication between neurons and groups of neurons.

Whereas without coherence, inputs arrive at random phases of the neuron excitability cycle and are much less effective in communicating. The shared resonance (synchronization) in a human brain achieves gamma synchrony, involving larger numbers of neurons and neuronal connections than is the case for beta or theta rhythms alone.

Unconditional compassion meditation produces high-amplitude gamma brainwave oscillations (20-40 Hz) which produce whole-brain-synchrony occurs particularly in the Prefrontal Lobe area. Meditators induce a sustained EEG high-amplitude gamma-band oscillations and phase-synchrony during objectless loving-kindness and compassion meditation. The gradual increase of gamma activity during meditation shows that neural synchronization is a network phenomenon that requires time to develop and prolonged practice improves efficiency, such that long-term meditators use less brain energy to maintain neural synchronization.

The inner/outer Janus of consciousness is composed of a neurological system that has three components: Afferent, Efferent, and Associative. Afferent—refers to the sensory side or processing of incoming information. Efferent—the motor or doing side, by which the nervous system manipulates one's own body and the outside world. Associative—or relating parts of the brain, refers to the sum total of internal processing of thoughts and feelings. There must be perfect cooperation within the inner self through the proper relation of energies to obtain self knowledge (Know Thyself) to apply the will in accord with the cosmic design, thereby realizing a cohesive relationship with the cosmos.

The psychic force of the subconscious radiates into conscious awareness, meaning the intuitive focus of the soul subjugates the physical to attune to Source via coherent sound at the Fibonacci frequency. Tesla maintained the integrity of his genius through the enhanced electromagnetic fields produced by his inventions, which he used to attune his intuitive psychic gnosis of meditative visualization and the reception of cosmic forces.

"The hadonic force probably is also the modus operandi behind the DNA molecular bonding stability, whilst being a composite entirely composed of the binomial triangle octave cascade of numbers instigated by 8hz electrolysis of water."
~ Ananda Bosman, www.akasha.de/~aton/HyperDNA.htm

PLUGGING IN

"The mind is sharper and keener in seclusion and uninterrupted solitude. No big laboratory is needed in which to think. Originality thrives in seclusion free of outside influences beating upon us to cripple the creative mind. Be alone, that is the secret of invention; be alone, that is when ideas are born. That is why many of the earthly miracles have had their genesis in humble surroundings."
~ Nikola Tesla

An individual that is not plugged into the cosmos is by default plugged into human culture without a compass, or buffer against the insanity of systemic exploitation and abuse. We learn slavitude as young children becoming compliant out of our need for attention and affection, then we go on as adults to sell ourselves short in one fashion or another to a rapacious machine that cares not for the individuals within its bounds. The cult of rank capitalism cares only for profit at the expense of nature and everything in its path.

In Borg culture the individual is a myth, for there are few true individuals within the four-dimensional Flatland of power, wealth, possessions and security. Security in all its forms is the main focus of a people whom are deprived of their sovereignty and dignity and their right to be unique. Not only do our thoughts not matter, neither do our emotions, our visions, our imagination and our truth.

In a socioeconomic world devoted to the accumulation of power as a denial of death and hedge against insecurity, there is no real community or long term planning...no sense of the human continuum moving into an evermore profound and amazing future. Individual gains in liberty and genius mean little when civilization itself is hitting the wall of its own hollow, shallow lack of HUmanness. Without a center, rooted into the cosmos, both the individual and the species has no integrity or sustainability...and instead becomes addicted to all forms of power advantage, through which a petty immortality project is substituted for the Mystery, magic and magnificence of being HUman.

"Until we evolve beyond the fetters of our own mistaken identity - until we can evolve from a consciousness of tyranny to a consciousness of consciousness - the idea of restoring balance to the world will remain no more than a half-baked fantasy."
~ *Philip Shepherd, 'New Self New World'*

Trying to spelunk into the internal world through mindfulness, self-reflection and meditation, when the body and mind are not keyed into the frequencies, strength and integrity of nature and Gaia — is like a form of self-torture. For if we are not plugged into the energies and information flow of the Universe prior to self and prior to humankind and our past conditioning, then all we have to bring to our self-awareness is layers upon layers of sickness, and we remain locked into a labyrinthian path that forever entraps the minotaur of our betrayal of our own existence.

By merging with the frequencies of nature we gain the integrity and beauty of nature at the deepest possible levels. Although it is seldom recognized, the drive to become more HUman is our principle drive. We become more HUman through cosmic sympathetic resonance or the sacred Music of the Spheres. HUmanization is autopoetic self-organization or cosmic illumination via the symphony of the Muse pouring forth from Source. The perfection of cosmic design requires the conscious intention of love through connecting to our true nature. The sovereign Muse expresses "passionate ambivalence" of the comedian. Critics and revolutionaries can easily get themselves killed when they speak the truth, while comics can get away with anything.

Imagine responding to people in a witty vignettes which electrify social interactions. We could create a practice of evolutionary social interaction instead of Borgsville speak, by building a fantastic generous inspired visionary mind. Humor increases the light...ie: HU-more. That is it makes us more HUman is the transcendent associative play of the prefrontal lobes which tickles the amygdala forward, as Neil Slade likes to say. In this way wisdom can "penetrate," whereas often the egoic defense and the collapse of the HUman into darkness prevents illumination of higher visionary perspectives.

Disenfranchisement goes hand in hand with usury societies because the spirit has to be broken in order to be intimidated, and only the disenfranchized, intimidated masochistic individual would submit themselves to abuse and to being bottom dog. Thus we have the commodification of the knowledge base and the wholesale collapse of practical commonsense and sensitivity to consequences. The point being that the habit of Borg culture is already so descended and retarded that we live in a falsely constructed gloom and doom world based on fear — whereas the transcendent reality is more akin to the way things really are — if we could only see clearly (hindsight, foresight, insight, oversight). HUmor helps us to see what already is.

The Sovereign is into the direct connection to Nature and into ephemeralized subtle technology as well. That is back to our hominid origins and into the galactic community. Back and forward, Up and Down, In and Out, Community and Individuality, Agency and Communion, into the Soma and the Psyche. Equally in all directions to expand the depth potential of Being. We have to go inside in order to get outside the box of the cul de sac of material reductionism. Phi is implicit in lifeforce, biogenic integrity, the Force, God, sustainability, eternity now, Timelessness.

Phi is optimization, such as in Mihály Csíkszentmihályi's positive psychology concept of the "Flow State" of perfect efficiency in performance. It is being in the Zone. https://www.flowgenomeproject.com/

DEEP LISTENING: Deep or active listening is a matter of fair-witness interoception by the inner senses of the body, rather than the confrontational, dismissive, competitive listening of the ego. The awareness of our emotions involves interoception — or the attention to internal bodily states. It is sometimes referred to as the "sixth sense" or Presence. Body awareness of our inner signals such as the heartbeat might lead to emotional awareness.

Freedom is the most basic law of life in the Universe, and only through freedom is there evolution under the Phi flow of Eros.

HOLY-HEALING-WHOLING

Drugs don't heal, only nature heals and makes whole. In fact healing doesn't heal or make whole. If sickness, disease and distress occur it is due to the inherited continuum of the civilizational environment that is causing it, which works against the full health and enlightenment of the individual. In order to be sovereign and recover cosmic-indigenous levels of health and wholism we must personally recover from the "fallen" nature of the human species itself.

All those things from Borg civilization that undermine our well-being must be transcended via meta-adaptation in order to overcome any and all illness. Under-adaptation, in reacting to a negative with negativity, inevitably increases entropy and chaos. We do everything to ourselves depending on our relationship in bringing the duality of polar reality into harmony. Health of the whole HUman can only be achieved by proper energy relationship with nature and the Universe.

The proper relation of energies refers to the Fibonacci ratio of frequencies, or the reverberatory formation of resonant standing waves forming a multi-frequency field of sympathetic resonance. **Georges Lakhovsky** in his book "*The Secret of Life*" tells us that living cells not only produce and radiate oscillations of very high frequencies, but they also receive and respond to oscillations imposed upon them from outside sources. When these outside sources of oscillations are in sympathetic resonance with the cell, the strength and vigor of that cell will be reinforced and become stronger. If on the other hand, these outside frequencies are of a different, dissonant frequency, compared to the cell's native oscillations, they might dampen or weaken them rather than reinforcing them, resulting in a loss of vigor and vitality for that cell.

Georges Lakhovsky was specifically talking about the ocean of cosmic rays or Tesla's idea of aether, however by "environmental oscillations" I am referring to cosmic frequencies from the sun, moon, planets and earth, the paramagnetic strength of the earth, the vitality of the soil, the lifeforce in our food, the biolophillic design of our architecture, the dralas or mana encompassed within our manmade landscapes and art, the frequencies given off by our machines, the élan vital embodied by living things, and the noospheric health composed of the mental-emotional activity of humans and other animals. Our physical, electromagnetic, social and cultural environment must be conducive to biological, mental and spiritual vitality for cosmic health and cosmic consciousness to be possible. Disease causing environments, disease causing organisms, and disease causing people, produce different frequencies than healthy cells and healthy people.

I am proposing a movement away from the unconscious animal power games, to a way of Being in which we can maximize our potential as humans... to Self actualize. This sense of transcending sadomasochism (dominance/submission) has to be bodily, mentally and spiritually Grokked. That is it cannot be simply a philosophical exercise or an idle wish. The body has to discover, recognize and remember its noble, "whole" condition and perpetuate the sovereign state regardless of interference. It takes conscious applied effort not to slip back into the automatic behavioral reactions in response to power-over chemistry. The first step is "self-validation" irrespective of worldly phenomena. Our future lies within us. Society will not change to be more life-positive until there is a change in the embodiment of our Humanity. Our resistance to a thing binds us to it. Indeed resistance is futile, transcendence is the key!

The big realization with the sovereignty work, was that negative power is cannibalistic, thus those still operating in the Hindbrain mode are predator/parasites. Whether they are attacking or seducing others they are literally spiritually and energetically eating them for their own security and sustenance. Obviously this form of energy relationship is unsustainable and fundamentally unethical in that it promotes disease and distress ubiquitously in everything that it touches. The "taking and usury" frequencies are anti-Golden Rule and are ultimately evolutionary selected against if order, health, beauty and abundance for all are to occur, and in this way civilization becomes more civilized. Only the Golden Rule truly supports life on earth!

The way forward doesn't require the exit the personal, but the of expansion the sense of the personal to include all fellow humankind, all life on earth and the Universe herself. The first step to transformation is to get stumped and flabbergasted over how impossible it is to proceed under the present species modus operandi. Then on going inside, and expanding our sense of self into limitless freedom — then the soul-utions arise from an Always Already archetypal perfection. We learn to create as the Universe creates, by becoming One with her. Any transgression against life sets us back from being Always Already Whole. Prior to trauma and the fallen state of the species, we hold the template for Platonic perfection within.

Don't compromise yourself for attention, acceptance or for the sake of media promotion or the applause of the crowd. The connoisseur doesn't compromise because he or she is always already OK. The hungry ghost races around looking for affection, attention, validation and meaning because the presovereign is an "outer-seeker," looking for succor and security in the world. But there is no outer-satiety for those with inner hunger, for inner-deficiency can never be met and filled from the outside, except under rare and sacred circumstances when the seeker has already done their work.

Become a destiny creator and quickly we realize that manifesting reality is an inside job. It is not that the outer world is "meaningless" it is just that "meaning" is something that only we can give to our existence through the **epicurious talent** of coming ALIVE to our sovereign Self. In order to give people back to themselves, we must first give our Self back to our selves. For we can't share the light, if we haven't already found it, and fanned the flames. What is our relationship to the energetic currency of life....the infinite Super Light of Spirit that animates our being?

Multidimensional abundance consciousness creates from an always already fullness and so every decision is satiated with satisfaction and gratitude.

CHAPTER 3

MASTER SOVEREIGNTY SERIES

"In the silence of our own darkness sparks a light - embodied with the presence of eternal peace it takes flight - from the heart we resonate the light of oneness in love for the sovereignty of all life." ~ Lee Parore

In order to relax you have to take the "noise" or static off the nervous system, because relaxation is coming into alignment, and "static" is the opposite of resonant coherence. The property of being coherent means a logical, orderly, and aesthetically consistent relationship of parts. The Core Supercharger, The Heart-tree Meditation and CardioMuscular Release are the most advanced practices for central nervous system defragmention through building the inner marriage ~ the balanced interchange of electromagnetic energy. The Heart-tree Meditation is the "hub" of sovereign practice that infuses all other practices with greater meaning and cuts through any social disharmony, subconscious terror or deviation from the path of truth. Opening the Mouth of God, Mito Meditation and the Blue Spot Meditation are the key Sovereignty Inner Arts for bodymind integration.

You can feel yourself growing new capacities even with a little Inner Arts practice and so you will have to remove stagnation in your life and change your environment to support that growth. By focusing on the enchanting beauty of heart-intelligence we find the master series of the sovereignty practices. When actively looking for the master series of sovereignty practices — I don't look outside, but inside. My work is the accumulation of about 13 years of this kind of exploration that I call the Inner Arts. I don't force the arrival of the practices, they come of their own volition by working on the blockage of the light that arises in me due to the pain of "social difficulty." They usually arrive autopoetically of their own accord while working on myself in bed after hours of sleeplessness.

Magically through substantiating the sovereign state we allow others to come into their own empowerment and freedom. Freedom is nowhere to be found in the looking outside for it. Sovereignty or freedom IS you! All conflicts in the outer world can be first resolved by unseizing the knots in the inner landscape. We are free when freeing all else. Freedom is achieved through letting go of the myopia of clinging and integrating higher levels of expansiveness. Real work is self-work for the soul has to be invited out of hiding. Only the true heart can pull the sword of Excalibur out of the stone. If we wait for someone else to do it for us, we will be waiting until the end of time.

When we are actively engaged in growth, we don't have time for stagnation, regression, defense, self-destruction and death.

CARDIOMUSCULAR RELEASE (CMR)

In 1997 I was massaging people in California and I found many would come to me with scattered brains. I asked myself how to get rid of brain scatter, because my brain would start resonating with their brains and thus it was irritating to work on scatterbrained people. A month went by and while working on myself n bed one night I did a three-step jumper-cable holding technique. As soon as I did it, I realized I had discovered the anti-scatter method I was looking for. The technique for getting rid of brain scatter I called Cardio Muscular Release (CMR).

CMR works on increasing the conscious and vibratory connection between the heart and the sympathetic trunk running either side of the spine on the neck and thorax. It is the only thing I have found to get rid of brain scatter and to unlock the neck and shoulders from the inside out. The heart is a hologram for the entire neuro-musculature of the body. CMR is a neurological jumper-cable technique using the heart as a holographic key to unlock the muscles of the neck and shoulders and to take the static off the nervous system. It entrains and relaxes the heart, breathing, metabolism and brain, unlocking the neuromuscular system from the inside out; as such it is way more effective, profound and lasting than massage.

CMR is a simple technique that opens the neck/shoulders/heart and turns off the fight-or-flight and removes static from the central nervous system so current/consciousness can flow with less friction and greater efficiency. CMR is very useful to move through any fear or resistance as our contraction becomes tangibly felt and we permanently melt into a progressively deeper sentient experience of our existence. This technique can be self-administered and is useful for improving concentration, to take the static off the nervous system, prior to meditation, headaches, processing emotions, insomnia, and to relieve muscle pain and tension. The effects are accumulative over time and will permanently rewire the nervous system from more primitive reptilian function toward a more spiritual and less reactive condition. Done as a daily practice it is both preventative and restorative.

Car crash victims and others with PTSD will find this technique invaluable for getting relief from an overactive sympathetic nervous system (HPA axis). When working on the muscles that are involved in the vigilance to danger—the neck, shoulders and jaw—I often find that electrical energy and spasms occur in the legs. Showing that the ego/socialization structure of the brain that is also associated with the vigilance muscles is inhibiting the full release of the charge from fight flight. Normally an animal would run after it comes out of its freeze response. We humans however do not remember to run off the charge generated by exposure to the tiger of daily existence.

Cardiomuscular Release (CMR) uses three holding positions on each side of the body and the heart is divided into three sections: 1. Left-top, 2. Right-top, 3. Bottom.

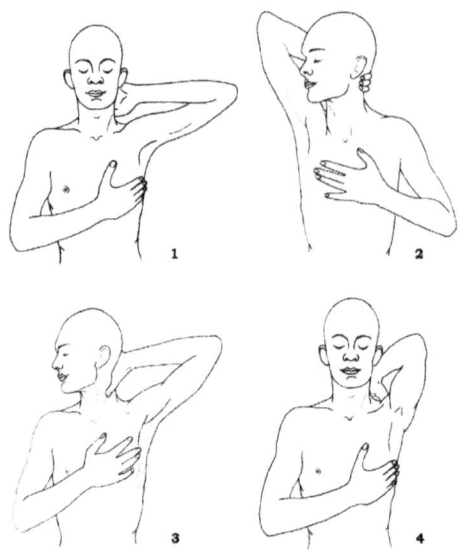

- **Position 1:** The three middle fingers of the left hand are placed along side left of the spine on the back of the neck; put fingertips onto the spine first and then pull off to the side to get good purchase on the ganglia. The right hand is placed on the left of the heart. Hold 5-10 minutes while throaty belly breathing.
- **Position 2&3:** The head is turned to the right, and the right hand reaches behind the neck and holds the left neck at the point where the sternocleidomastoid muscle joins the skull just under the left ear. Left hand is on the right-side of the heart at the middle of the chest. Hold 5 minutes while throaty belly breathing.
- **Position 4:** The left hand reaches up over the shoulder and down the back and the fingers poke into the Erector spinæ muscles alongside the spine between the scapulars. The right hand is on the bottom of the heart. While throaty belly breathing slide left hand slowly up the spine over the course of 10 minutes.

Repeat all three positions in mirror fashion on the other side of the body as well for a full release to occur, otherwise one will continue to feel some static and disconnection. Remain present and sensitive throughout the process and hold each position until you get the AHA. Meditation, Toning, the Inner Smile and dropping the back of the tongue can be done along with CMR.

By taking the static off the nervous system the brain is fed by a stronger more coherent flow of energy by which it may command and optimize the body.

PSYCHOSPACIAL MEDITATION

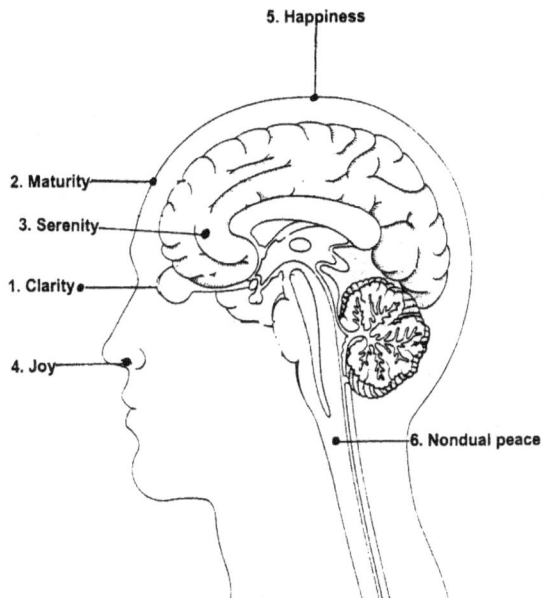

If one focuses the Mind's-Eye in a directional spacial orientation:
1. **Clarity**—occurs as a single-point in front of the two eyes.
2. **Maturity**—is at the top of the forehead.
3. **Serenity**—is at the temporal lobes above the ears.
4. **Joy**—is found by focusing the mind's-eye at the nostrils and following the breath there.
5. **Happiness**—(the absence of closure and sadness) is found by focusing at the crown of the head and this lifts sadness in the lungs/throat/diaphragm.
6. **Nondual Peace**—After running through the full sequence then a painful knot of "need" is felt in the solar plexus. This knot in the solar plexus is then dissolved by focusing the mind's-eye on the brainstem. By practicing clarity, maturity, serenity and joy all at the same time; this then translates as peace.

Psychospacial Meditation is like a gate opener for connecting the Uraeus, the brainstem and the solar plexus brain. These psychospacial gateways allow the knot of need/control in the solar plexus to be accessed and dissolved by first passing through clarity/maturity/serenity/joy/happiness and then finally this control-knot is "touched" and healed through the "brainstem." So perhaps final letting go of the reactive distress of our separation and unenlightenment is done in this way. When we are talking of resistance, division, judging, distancing etc... we are probably talking about feeling helpless or the "need to control." So this is the tension that prevents Unity Consciousness and harmony with our environment.

Interestingly the pain and deficit in the solar plexus knot was not apparent to awareness until I had done all the focus points. However this knot must subliminally always be there as a permanent ongoing wound. I theorize that if one clears the larger-noisier emotions out the way, the finer more nuanced emotions would be felt and one's inner life should deepen and refine, becoming ever more precise in communicating subtle emotional resonances and information from the Void.

I intuit that the sequence is important. Clarity is necessary prior to maturity. Maturity is necessary prior to serenity. Serenity is necessary prior to joy. Joy is necessary prior to happiness. Happiness is necessary prior to overcoming deprivation/need. Thus there is a specific flow to the unfolding of energy in the body. Psychospacial meditation will permanently rewire one if done consistently. Individual reasons and issues for suffering are not important, it's a matter of rewiring and changing the vibratory state of the tissues. Thus all hurts are one, and all healing is one.

The key to psychospacial meditation: I found the sequence to the psychospacial gates by simply by holding the word in my mind and seeing where my mind's-eye went. This way we should be able to find the psychospacial focal point for any such word, eg: forgiveness, fortitude, gratitude, benevolence etc.... Focus your mind's-eye on any pain, constriction or ill feeling in the body and ask "what is this?" After a while a word will arise reflecting the dominant emotion connected with that blockage in the flow. Then find the opposite word and send the mind's-eye on a hunt to search for the location and the mechanism that switches the stuck negative emotion into its opposite resonance. In this way we can shift any vibration over to the positive. By emotionally spring cleaning in this way we do not have to remain victim to entrenched, stressful states that play havoc with our health and well-being.

• **V FOR HUMOR**—Dopamine is a neurotransmitter that regulates movement, balance, emotion and motivation, and it also stimulates the pleasure reward centers of the brain. I found the Psychospacial Technique for increasing dopamine and norepinephrine in the prefrontal lobes to increase humor, improve mood and provide social immunity. While your eyes are closed, focus the mind's eye into a V shape, extending from the top of your nose and up into your forehead and extend the V into antennae sticking out the top of your head above the eyes. This increases consciousness and blood flow to the region, and promotes spontaneous good humor, lightness and mood change. Humor is the best way to transcend Borg shaming, intimidation and limitation mechanisms of sinning, guilting, shoulding and holier than thou. Humor is associated wtih prefrontal lobe activity that probablydown regulates the amygdala also. Even if you have to do HA.HA.HA.HA type chanting and jumping jacks to get the humor juices flowing, eventually you will cultivate a more humorous attitude and altitude about life.

Dopamine enhancing herbs will greatly help with free flowing humor: Mucuna, Bala, Ginkgo Biloba. Curcumin. Oregano Oil. ginseng, nettles, red clover, enugreek, dandelion and peppermint, Magnesium. Green Tea. Vitamin D. Sunflower, pumpkin, milk thistle, chia and hemp seeds also boost dopamine and norepinephrine levels.

HEART-TREE MEDITATION

The Heart is the ultimate metaphor for point-of-use technology, in that the more that it is encouraged, the more the heart reveals itself to us.

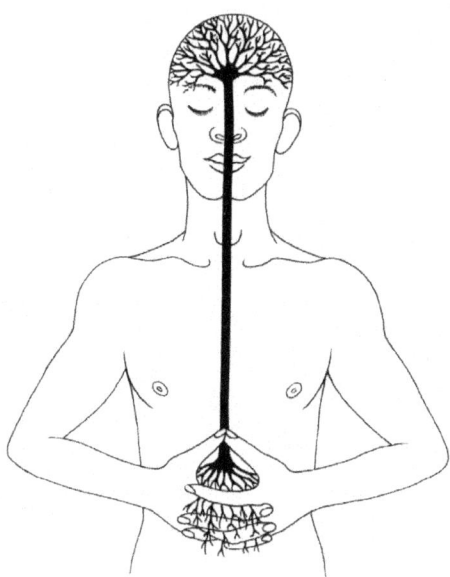

The root of the word courage is "*cor*" is the Latin word for heart. The Heart-Tree Meditation is the most profound practice for calming Borg-distress, or eliminating inner/outer Borg energies. So far this is the principle meditation for building up the higher mammalian spindle cell network, ie: the apex of emotional integration of body-mind-soul. While lying in bed (or on the earth) interlace your fingers and cup your hands at the solar plexus near the bottom of the sternum with the sense that you are holding the root ball of the Heart-tree. Drop the tongue into the belly and cease thought by feeling into the heart, and now build the trunk of the tree extending into your head.

Then look up with your eyeballs and pull your Mind's Eye into the canopy of the brain and see-feel a branched tree reaching up into the prefrontal cortex and crown. Feel "light" moving through the branches of the brain canopy while feeling the roots of the Heart-tree in your solar plexus amplified by your interlocked hands. As you do this you are setting up a resonant field from the heart direct to the spindle network, thereby greatly feeding the sovereign self with the nectar of conscious elevated presence. You will need to breathe deeply and slowly to maintain your grip on this high-energy state. Toning HUM with the mouth closed releases the diaphragm (roots) and energizes and cleans the spindle cell brain canopy (shoots).

While lying down the legs must be either straight or gently raised with a pillow under the knees. Hands can be clasped higher up on the chest or lower on the solar plexus to widen the territory for the seat of the heart, relieve blockage and increase coherent, sympathetic resonance—and present a different octave for the brain charging. When establishing the whole tree you need to look into the canopy with your eyeballs, and your mind's eye. This pulls energy from your solar plexus roots, so that the whole tree becomes one. The solar plexus (serotonin, 8 Hz) enteric brain is the roots of the head brain, without establishing a tacit-sensorial link between the two brains, the brain hemispheres become divided and our betawave adaptive consciousness becomes divorced from our heart, emotions and mystical right-brain.

"Only one or two thousand nerve fibers connect the brain to the hundred million nerve cells in the small intestine. Those hundred million nerve cells are quite capable of carrying on nicely, even when every one of their connections with the brain is severed..." Dr. Michael D. Gershon, the author of "The Second Brain"

After the solar plexus root ball and tree is firmly established you can bring your hands down to the lower belly and put the thumb-steeple at the navel. Build another root ball, longer trunk and canopy. This incorporates the entire viscera into the governance of the beneficent brain. But it also heals the pelvic area to support full integrity/integration or whole consciousness.

When you look at the caustic effects of social terror and stress on the bodymind, it is no wonder we are so operationally retarded — compared to our vast potential. A stable connection to Source is our only real security, protection and happiness. The faster and deeper we rewrite our operating system the more confidence and momentum we have in changing the world around us. The Heart-tree Meditation quickens the incarnation of spirit through a mainline feeding of the higher emotional integrating circuits, thus the Heart-tree meditation is a principle method of reconnecting with Presence and overcoming self-abandonment. You may find your Borg self trying to fight you for attention, but just drop whatever drama it tries to regurgitate and go back always to this primary linkup of the heart, the canopy of spindle cells and prefrontal lobes (Uraeus or the *all seeing eye*). Wherever the individual's ATTENTION so goes his power.

Do this meditation daily along with the Light Sword and Uraeus Meditation and Royal Jelly for the fastest route to sovereignty and a deep, grounded sense of wholeness and well-being. With regular Heart-tree Meditation the niggling issues of mundane reality disappear into the peace, love and harmony of indescribable unity. Once proficient at holding the mind's eye at the tree branches that feed the neocortex, you may be able to do an eyes open Heart-tree Meditation while engaged in upright walking. In this way the alpha and the omega of the sovereignty practices can be joined into one very powerfully connecting practice. Don't get stuck in rebellion, but slide quickly over to celebration, for only that generates cerebralization.

If a pelvic floor contraction (Kegel) is done with each deep breath during the Heart-tree meditation, this perineum bandha effect sends a wave of light up the body to light up the Heart-tree in association with the breath, thereby pulse lighting up the oxygenated Heart-tree in rhythmic movement from its roots to its shoots. This is the Christmas tree or Christos, the inner anointing of the inner Light. The Merkaba is an antigravity starship.

• HEART-EYES MEDITATION

You can capital-eyes on the high-contact, quality connected felt-sense you have built up in the solar plexus through the Heart-tree meditation to generate more loving, radiant and attractive eyes. As you go through your day, it is possible to observe how open and loving people's hearts are through their eyes. The cooperation, order, cocreativity, good-will and community feeling created is catalyzed by the heart's power to communicate and effect change through the eyes. After you have done the Heart-Tree Meditation keep one hand on the solar plexus and the other on your eyes. Set up a felt-resonant connection between the solar plexus, the heart and eyes.

In order to access your inner kinesthetic sense you will need to apply the three keys: Dropping the muscles at the back of the tongue, doing an inner smile and a throaty breath. After you have built up your neurology of Love Eyes it is just a matter of remembering to soften your eyes and facial muscles throughout the day, especially when around other people.

We are rapidly undoing ourselves and awakening beyond all we have known ourselves to be and our "reactions" to how we think things are. Resistance to our own liberation and happiness is all that holds us back from ever expanding integration and fruition. Heart by heart conscious expansion will prevail because of the very weight of spiritual development already inherent within our collective makeup. This flowering will inevitably spread both through the media, person to person and morphogenically via the noosphere. We are being given new eyes to see.

"Courage is not the absence of fear. It is acting in spite of it." ~ Mark Twain

• FOUNT OF HAPPINESS

In the Psycho-Spacial Meditation happiness is a fountain of light through the core of the brain and pouring out of the crown. So when doing the Core Supercharger you can feel this column of energy rising from the bliss dish of the jaw (Inner Smile). Happiness is the builder, guardian and protector of the immune system. Happiness is a prerequisite to focus, and Source is the force of focus. The Fount of Happiness is the purifying elixir — the laser that organizes matter into coherent order, allowing a perfected high efficiency brain, capable of supernatural feats. With apriori happiness we have the strength to not delve into stressful thought, emotions or behaviors, therefore we do not accumulate the stressful energies of entropy and decay that lead to maladaptive behaviors. Thus we can "build" to gain lift off speed against the gravity and inertia of material existence, to live our magical essence—being knowledgeable, emotionally aware, self-directed, and at peace with the world. Hubris makes reality satirical, but to the sovereign "the facts are friendly," thus they accept reality more than most people, see through phoniness, lies and games, and they deal with problems rather than avoid them, and forgive shortcomings—hence relax into Being.

Positive emotional tone is an inside job, as we cannot rely on the complex, changing world to "cause" us happiness, joy and love.

•HAPPY HIPPOCAMPUS MEDITATION

The Happy Hippocampus Meditation is a surefire way to manufacture happiness from within. The Hippocampus is located on the floor of each lateral ventricle of the brain, thought to be the center of emotion, memory, and the autonomic nervous system. The shape of the elongated ridges looks like a seahorse and is depicted as such in art, most often as a horse with a mermaid tail. The Happy Hippocampus meditation can be done lying in bed, on one's stomach with your head on its side, so that the arms and pillow arrangements allow support for you to press your dominant thumb onto your Third Eye.

Then you do The Three Kings (Inner smile, Tongue drop, Throaty breath) and feel into your Hippocampus. Essentially imparting happiness into your Hippocampus with your meditation focus. Lying on your back and putting a piece of shungite on your Third Eye while meditating greatly amplifies the meditative function and results. You will have to repeat the word "Happiness" while you do this, because your inner Hippocampus seahorse is probably pretty unhappy and so you have to apply consciousness into it order to change its vibratory state and emotion, while pressing firmly into the Third Eye You may notice resistance to the happiness vibration change in your Hippocampus because this meditation uncovers the depth of death, sadness, loss, deprivation and unhappiness we harbor within our brain, however if we don't apply ourselves to brain change, we may go through life in deep dissatisfaction and grief with no means of changing our life circumstances to bring us joy. Once you are able to easily activate the Happy Hippocampus, the meditation can be done while sungazing for added rewiring/frequency change; or using a piece of Shungite on the third eye to help wipe the slate clean and energize. Often with need various "assists" to palpate, touch and transform numb, comatose or insensate, inactive regions of the brain. Regular exercise releases endogenous opioids, enhances serotonin function, stimulates nerve growth factors, promotes cell proliferation in the hippocampus, and leads to a livelier, better-oxygenated brain. BTW the more alcohol that one drinks the more atrophy occurs in the brain's memory storing hippocampus.

•HYPOTHALAMUS ASSURANCE BOOST

After you have generated happiness in the Hippocampus, you will need to generate "reassurance" in the Hypothalamus which the Hippocampus connects into. While meditating - look back through the optic nerve into the brain core and send reassuring light into the Hypothalamus. The Hypothalamus is region in the central core of the brain that coordinates both the autonomic nervous system and the activity of the pituitary, controlling body temperature, thirst, hunger, and other homeostatic systems, and involved in sleep and emotional activity.

As social animals our sense of "security" or self-affirmation is socially generated, however in the competitive Borg society we are more likely to receive negative or subversive feedback which atrophies or starves our Hypothalamus...that is, our autonomic emotional regulator. As you focus your attention on the Hypothalamus send into it the light of reassurance while mentally repeating a supportive word such as comfort, encouragement, assistance, sustenance, help, relief, goodness, wholeness etc...

• GOODIFYING EMEDITATION

This is one of the most important Inner Arts because if we cannot generate good feelings from within, we are vulnerable to the outer world determining our inner state. The Goodifying Emeditation (the "E" stands for emotional) overcomes the disenfranchisement caused by self-rejection and rejection from others. It is this toxic inheritance which is the main interference pattern to a sovereign command of one's life, and is the seed energy for all our methods of self-abuse, self-sabotage and self-negation. So first you need to get into the body to "operate it" and to do that do the Three Kings (tongue drop, throaty breath, inner smile).

Then in relaxed meditation, look back into the brain as though the forehead was a spotlight, you will focus feeling directly into the judicial center, ie: the *anterior cingulate cortex* and corpus callosum. You may feel an unfathomable hunger in this area, as though it is bruised and needy. As you breathe into the neediness and focus the mind's light on this area, repeat the word "Goodness" and self-absolve yourself of any sin implicated onto you by the unlawful, selfish needs of others. As you shine the mind's eye through the forehead, into the core of the brain, you will notice that the Adam's Apple area of the throat starts to pulsate in unison with the diaphragm. This is a rhythmic orgasm of sorts that arises from the Goodifying focused energy of the brain meeting the opened grateful heart. You know you have made contact with the limbic brain and brainstem when you see a warm golden red glow inside your brain core.

The Goodifying Emeditation can be practiced in bed, or lying on the grass, and can also be incorporated into sungazing sessions, baths, bus rides, or walking etc... If you sit by the rapids of a river, with your bare feet on the ground or in the water. The negative ions from the rapids acts to enhance the field force of your meditation and facilitate rapid healing/wholing. There is significant immune enhancement via doing the Goodifying emeditation near river rapids. I was doing the Goodifying Emeditation down by the river and noticed increased warmth/chi under the jaw as the immune system gets a boost, reflecting the increased tantric-yogic action of being around high negative ion sources. Homes, yoga studios and temples need to be built around high negative ion generating sources in nature.

The Goodifying Emeditation is the most advanced Inner Art I have found yet...as it allows us to vibrationally break the hexing and spells of the various trauma and abuses against us. Plus depending on our attachment style to our parents...Goodifying our brain allows us to heal the various insults to our sovereign core and gain the detachment necessary to be our own person. That is by recognizing and appreciating our own self we free ourselves from the deprivation and neediness of codependent Borg society, and our addiction to ongoing abuse. Responding to a transgression against us in a "sovereign" way is like good parenting—we take the energy that would have gone into the primitive victim-victor cycle and take response-ability in the moment for a favorable outcome.

Overcoming the inner conflict and the war of opposites allows all parts of our whole to integrate, conjunct and cohere, that is to make love, to BE Love!

NEUROEMOTIONAL REPROGRAMMING

Neuroemotional Reprogramming (NER) is allowing, resetting and fine tuning the body's vibrational resonance, in order to grow the neurochemistry and neurons (dendrites) for the Universal bodymind. NER enhances the embodiment or incarnation of transcendental spiritual qualities/states such as peace, empowerment, worthiness, gratitude, trust, faith, reverence and equanimity. In the stepped down nature of our daily lives we often do not get to experience the conditions needed to spontaneously generate these higher vibrational states. Therefore we need a "daily practice" whereby our bodymind becomes trained and accustomed to generating these frequencies.

NER PRACTICE SEQUENCE: To rectify modern dissociative psychosis (ie: the emotional plague) the linear chakra system is turned upside down into belly with neuroemotional reprogramming. **Chakra-1.** Red-spleen-worthiness, **Chakra-2.** Orange-liver-gratitude, **Chakra-3.** Yellow-solar plexus-trust, **Chakra-4-5.** Green/Blue-Hara-Faith, **Chakra-6-7.** Indigo/Violet-above pubis-reverence/equanimity. Qualities are pulled into the heart on the in-breath then sent down to the area of the belly on the out-breath. The cosmic umbilical IS sympathetic resonance with the harmony of the spheres.

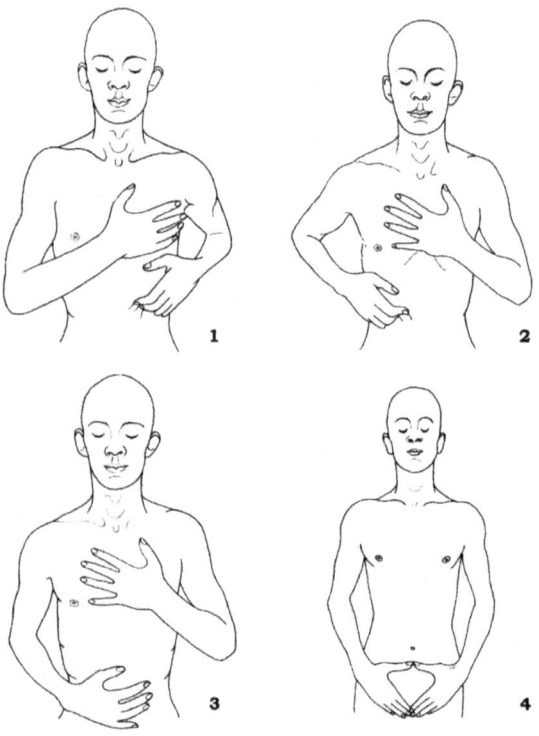

1• **Worthiness**—Put the left hand on the bottom of the left rib cage and push your fingers into the spleen. Place the right hand between the breasts on the right side of your heart. Hold this position while breathing worthiness in through the heart and pushing worthiness down into the spleen on the out breath. Worthiness-receptivity gives us the foundation or the correct stance (Kokoro-gamae) to be empowered to act in ways that build self-esteem. "Worthiness" represents a cellular level of YES to life without which we cannot fully incarnate, nor can we maintain a strong immune system, good health and receive or actualize the Self.

2• **Gratitude**—Change hands to cup the right-hand at the bottom of the right rib cage and push your fingers into the liver. Place the left hand between the breasts on the right side of your heart. The liver is the area that should be infused with Gratitude from the heart during attitudinal breathing. Gratitude links the brain directly to the enteric brain thereby giving us access to the "power" to take full responsibility for our lives. Feel into the generous quality of Gratitude pouring forth from the heart and send it down into the liver. This turns on the parasympathetic nervous system, and you might notice your digestion making noises. The liver must be bought into the fire of Gratitude first before Trust is real, for trust is born of gratitude. You have got to have biological trust and faith in order to open to fuller incarnation and empowerment; so we do not have to burn so much wasted energy in defense and resistance (mask, shield, ego).

3• **Trust**—Again holding the right side of the heart with one hand the other is placed on the solar plexus; which is the seat of power (sufficiency) and need (deficiency). Do the attitudinal breathing in through the heart and infuse the solar plexus with Trust. The trust we are generating here is not a circumstantial trust, but a Divine Trust, a cellular biological-trust beyond conditions. A sense of trust felt prior to differentiation, concept and distinction, prior to mind all together. This is not about trusting others or trusting life or even yourself. Wisdom and will, twined in One, issue forth from the solar plexus (soul-center) as rays from the sun. Trust through the solar plexus draws its power from the Great Unseen, whereby we build a deeper cellular connection to the All, free of contraction and fear.

• **Faith**—Jumper-cable with your hands between the right side of the heart and the lower Tantien, (the Hara, 2 inches below the navel area) and proceed with attitudinal breathing for Faith in this region. Faith is one of the last things approached in the neuroemotional sequence, as the final letting go into nothing. With the influx of faith into the lower belly you body should start feeling an antigravity effect. This work to establish biological faith is the direct door to Witness or Pure-Context Awareness.

4• **Reverence and Equanimity**—Pure Awareness, the marriage of intellect and intuition, is cultivated with the last neuroemotional step. Touch the thumbs together at the navel and create a diamond shape with your hands with fingertips touching the pubic bone. Generate a plasma ball of Reverence and Equanimity, thus growing the immovable seat of soul. Equanimity breathing and the generation of the Reverence Power-ball in the lower belly allow us to build a spiritual nervous system that is transcendent of the pros and cons and the twists and turns of life in order to bring our Realization effectively into the world through spiritual action. Without reverence and equanimity we are still driven by poverty consciousness, ie: inadequacy, deprivation, need, powerlessness and lack of harmony.

With this meditative therapy not only do we make up for the absence of emotional and spiritual nourishment during our developmental years, but after our NER conditioning is stabilized to higher emotional resonance, we find that our lives change in direct correspondence to the new resonant frequencies we embody. We thus radiate higher spiritual dominion both in our own behavior, thought, attractiveness, and in our energetic influence over the behavior and responses of others that come in contact with us.

So few of us were given a sense of self-worth and spiritual validation as a child that we live with a subliminal wrenching wound which we try and fill up by many different inferior tactics. NER takes us directly to Ground Zero, where we can be "organically receptive" to reconstruction into a higher estate. We stop fidgeting with our wound and open to the dominion of the Christ/Buddha within. Neuroemotional reprogramming is simply addressing the void in our socioemotional make up and building up our neurological structures to facilitate a deeper more meaningful life.

Through transcendental training via NER we grow the neuro-anatomy or esoteric anatomy for increasingly "universal boundaries." Thus we take on more of a species or global Being, and waste far less energy indulging in, enforcing and defending our smallness. Modern man doesn't know it yet, but emotional development and felt-Presence is the key to enlightened life and to enlightenment, because that is where we are most lacking.

We cannot expect to find, nor will we be given our higher spiritual qualities from the outside world. We must look within for the qualities of Clarity, Maturity, Serenity, Joy, Happiness, Peace, Empowerment, Worthiness, Gratitude, Faith, Trust, Reverence and Equanimity. These are aspects of the "Absolute" that we are attempting to integrate, they are not "Relative" or related to the conditioned worldly realm. These "inner qualities" cannot be derived by external means. If we do not find these qualities by internal means then the social world will seem indeed to be constantly undermining us, because we are expecting it to give us these qualities, and of course it never will—humanity has not yet reached the point of social reinforcement of Divinity as a daily occurrence.

If we did not grow up in ideal social conditions we have to grow the wiring for these Universal value qualities. If as a baby we were not given a sense of welcome, worth and value our spirit shied away from incarnating. Without biological self-worth we have no biological trust, and without trust we cannot establish biological faith. Without biological faith we cannot maintain a sustained sense of unity with all creation or God—with this emotional reprogramming method we find the void and invite in healing Presence.

In the externalized, usury world of material capitalism that exemplifies our current era, chances are our parents didn't even have the self-esteem or deep spiritual value qualities to give to us. So we cannot really blame them for not giving us that which they did not even have for themselves. It is after all the pain of this Self-betrayal that propels us forth on the hero's journey of Self-discovery. Thus humanity proceeds in awakening both from that love which it does acquire and from that which it still lacks. As that which has been unconscious suddenly becomes conscious, often the first response is fear. Transmutation involves taking that fear and transforming it through gratitude, reverence and equanimity into Pure Awareness.

The wholesale blockage of spiritual visionary consciousness is why our current civilization is hitting the wall with virtually no foot on the brakes. Asking questions and eliciting desire for soul-utions is where kundalini awakening and visionary downloads begins. Our job as cocreators of culture is to create psychobiological conditions in which futurevoyance is more likely to occur. Revealing "What Is," is the way of the sovereign, the sage, the shaman or the Jedi. Ask yourself questions, and your body will give you the answers. If you then do what it says, after a while you will have more questions and more answers, and so we learn how to wake up and come back to life from the inside out. The Inner Arts are an infinite revelation of the true nature of being HUman.

Enlightenment, empowerment, dropping of the pain-body and peace are a self-loving phenomenon. It is in the embodiment of biological self-esteem that our true self worth lays. Dropping of the bodymind is synonymous with "receptivity" and this in turn is synonymous with "worthiness." Essentially this is done by being at Absolute Peace (Ground Zero) long and deep enough to let the life within us grow and flow. When we actively affirm ourselves we green light our bodymind beyond the need for armoring ourselves against a sense of unworthiness. When you take the lid off of Pandora's box the stuff inside is no longer scary. We live partial lives to the degree that we keep the lid on. Thanatos or the death urge is a response to frustrated and blocked desire (Eros) that cannot grow and refine because it is repressed, and so that which is Good, True and Beautiful turns into its demonic, rather than daemonic form. This is why the human species is so destructive, because it has not been allowed to freely grow.

Power from Peace—Worthiness from Power—Presence from Worthiness—Gratitude from Presence—Trust and Faith from Gratitude—Reverence and Equanimity from Trust and Faith.

PRIMAL RELEASE POSE

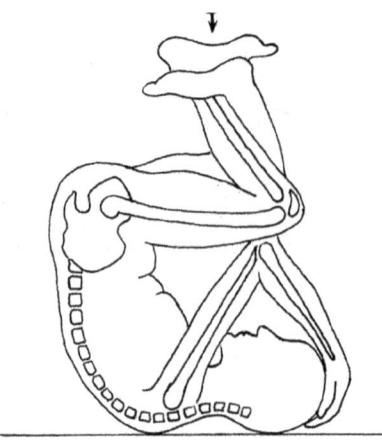

This pose is ideal for contemplating our "Fundamental Doubt" over whether the Universe is indeed supportive of us. Primal Release Pose addresses two of the major blocks in the body armor. The two areas in the bodymind where the reins on our spirit are pulled most tightly by the ego's entrenched defenses: The diaphragm and the Iliopsoas muscle complex. Opening these two muscles along with the rhomboids is essential to surrender into the heart expansion that constitutes spiritual life. If we can release these, we can free ourselves from the crippling effects of trauma, denial and the accumulation inner and outer negativity.

It is these two somatic blocks that lead to the unconsciousness and inertia resulting from dissociation. Since these blockages are set up in order to curb emotion, we cannot be emotionally authentic without opening up these two neuromuscular areas...and in doing so the Heart is then given preeminence in our psyche. This primal contraction release for the lower body involves contorting the body in a yogic pose to compress the diaphragm and psoas, waiting for an emotional discharge to occur, then breathing and pressing into the muscular spasm that occurs when the pose is dropped.

1. Warm up: First lie on your back, and gently pull your legs over your head taking care to avoid straining your neck muscles. Knees lightly bent, legs in the air. Put your weight on your thoracic/shoulder area, cup your hands over the crown of your head and rock back and forward, pulling gently on the head to extend the neck, thus rolling the spine into the floor. The spine will probably give a chiropractic adjustment or two..

2. Upsidedown Pose: Cross your feet in the air and place your elbows on your thighs about 4" above knees, while still holding the head and rest in this position with maximum body weight on the shoulders. Put all the weight from the legs directly down in a line of gravity to the shoulder girdle. Breathe deeply and stay in this position, gently wiggling around as desired for up to 10 minutes.

3. Enforced Spasm: Then lie flat on your back, holding the muscles of the small of the back, either side of the spine with the fingers splayed out. After a minute these muscles will spasm after having been over extended in the pose position. Press into the spasm with fingers and breathe into the belly until it subsides. The more one does the exercise the less spasms will occur. If spasms are too much to handle, lift knees to relax spine and press into spasms with fists.

This technique provides a gentle cathartic release of stored charge from the muscles. The discharge is interesting its like a rolling wave of energy-emotion coming from the diaphragm, often associated with a contemporary thought of sadness or self pity, however the thought is only what the psyche is using as a vehicle for the discharge to happen. The more this is done, the more the diaphragm is released and this straightens the spine and softens the belly allowing full breath. The PRP releases chronic contraction in the lumbar muscles — the innermost layer of these being the psoas. This contraction and release allows more space inside, and more conductivity through the pelvis and into the legs, better grounding and more connection between the top half and the lower half of the body. This pose is excellent for "getting stuff to the surface." So we could call this pose the upside-down insight-out pose.

The more clean, vitalized and disarmored we become the greater cosmic connection, and the less interference vibration from the Borg world affects us. By becoming whole or sovereign we gain immunity from the Borg. Kundalini naturally pools and builds where we are conditioned to stagnate due to various traumas or deficiencies in our past. It essentially creates a cauldron of heat and pressure there the body armor is concentrated due to some habitually unprocessed emotion (shame, guilt, fear, envy, self-hate, anger, futility, confusion). This focus of psychic energy in blocked areas can come from our own experience, from family psychosomatic conditions and habits and also from our ancestral line. You could say that those individuals that do not clear and release their body armor in their lifetime, pass it on to subsequent generations — and indeed affect everyone they meet for better or worse with their energetic field.

In this way body armor and PTSD is contagious through epigenetics, through EMF field resonance, through the noosphere, Psi-scalar-faster than light, as well as voice and emotions and thought, word and deed. Trauma you could say has a greater ripple effect than love or joy, because the subconscious takes more vigilant notice of threat and danger than of happiness and openness. To move the energy through a blocked area this takes inquiry as to the reasons for the damming up of Flow, Inner Arts mindful attention, touch and breath into the area. The blockage illuminates us as to its cause. Physical detoxification, perhaps including successive water fasting, and all manner of earthing, movement, stimulation, exercise and vibration helps to wake up the contracted/numb/tired/sleeping parts of ourselves.

The sovereign is nothing if not causal with regards to their lens of perception and their response.

THE INNER CANDLE MEDITATION

Compassion, the Fair Witness, and the Uraeus is the overlord function of the sovereign (the Übermensch—overman or superman) whereby we stop wasting energy in self/other judgment, rejection and blame. When you understand the human condition, there is no one to blame anyways, so forgiveness is not applicable. Perhaps the best brain-wipe for getting rid of blame/guilt/shame is the Inner Candle. By sending a rush of energy through the core of the brain we can erase the stuck record of hurt/blame tapes and self-righteous indignation in our judicial center the tissue around the corpus callosum—the **Anterior Cingulate Cortex** (ACC).

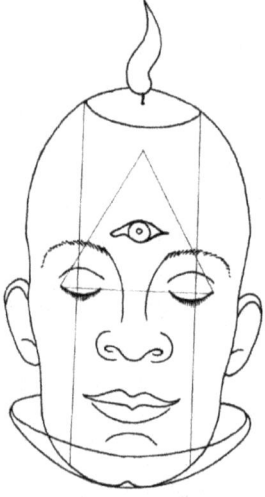

"The light of the body is the eye: if therefore thine eye be single, thy whole body shall be full of light." Jesus the Christ, Matthew 6:22

Do the Inner Smile, while feeling the jaw as a curved dish. On this dish imagine a 3" diameter candle rising as a column through the brain. With lids closed turn your eyeballs up at the top of your head to observe the flame of the imaginary candle. Inner Candle is like a force field of strength and uplift that can be done throughout the day, even while walking, in the bath or anytime as a method of generating Presence and a priori happiness. You can generate a permanent Inner Candle, remembering to look skyward, eyes open, to feed on the light and glory of your own being.

The Inner Candle is immediate restorative justice that resets and harmonizes the attraction/aversion judgment center, the Anterior Cingulate Cortex (ACC). The people's court is the lower ACC, while the Supreme Court is the upper ACC in association with the prefrontal lobes. By cleaning out the stored charge from past abuse, conflict, humiliation, injustice and rejection we can proceed without the fragmentation caused by the perseveration of shock-stress. Perseveration means prolonged response after the stimulus has ceased. In particular the Inner Candle in association with the Core Super Charger produces a regime change in the core of our worldview.

One of the signs that we still have work to do in defusing our Agency Court Center (ACC) is the sense of *double bind*, which disempowers forward movement due to the pervasive sense of Fucked-if-you-do/Fucked-if-you-don't! It is the brain's central court — the anterior cingulate cortex that governs fairness, jurisprudence, justice, rightness and goodness. A double bind is an emotionally distressing dilemma in which an individual receives two or more conflicting messages, so that no matter which directive is followed, the response will be construed as incorrect. The need to be "right" makes fools of us all, while the need to "BE" gets lost in the neurosis of endless manipulation, control and effort.

To work through the double binds and impossible dilemmas associated with family/work/romance — it is a matter of raising your own energy, grounding, aerobics, movement and actively following your Muse vocation. The double bind is a spanner in the neurological works that ultimately leads to hopelessness, depression and fatigue, so it is best to push into it by putting a more concerted effort into self care and your true life's work. Not everyone can see things on our level, nor operate on our level of morality and integrity…so if others cannot handle a greater truth we have to leave them to their own devises and move on to shining horizons.

• COMPLEX INNER CANDLE MEDITATION

The Inner Candle can be done while on your back listening to binaural music with ear phones on…and you can do the mind-meld pressure lock with both thumbs at the outer eye sockets and the index fingers together in a triangle at the top of the forehead. Again remember to let the body go into complete jellyfish state.

•THE REPTILE AND THE BUTTERFLY

You can voluntarily turn on the parasympathetic nervous system by lowering the jaw via dropping the tongue progressively into the belly. Then if you focus peace with the mind's eye on the brainstem and this turns off recriminations-defense mind that is associated with flight-fight chemistry. As the parasympathetic switches on the digestive and growth functions then are activated and the excited fear charge in the solar plexus disappears so that Trust may be built in that area.

Presence does not incarnate without this biological Trust being established in the solar plexus, and only through Presence is soul-relationship possible. We normally associate the more human-humane nurturing qualities with growth/parasympathetic/visceral activity. The activating or sympathetic nervous system's defense and protection mode doesn't allow for bonding and togetherness, nor "depth" in relationship. Learn how to connect with joy in the solar plexuses and you begin to live the noble sovereign life, in touch with your freedom and power.

THE URAEUS

The Uraeus is the sovereign's cosmic umbilical cord, which the ancient Egyptians showed us is the etheric field protruding from the anterior frontal lobes at the hairline—like the head of a cobra.

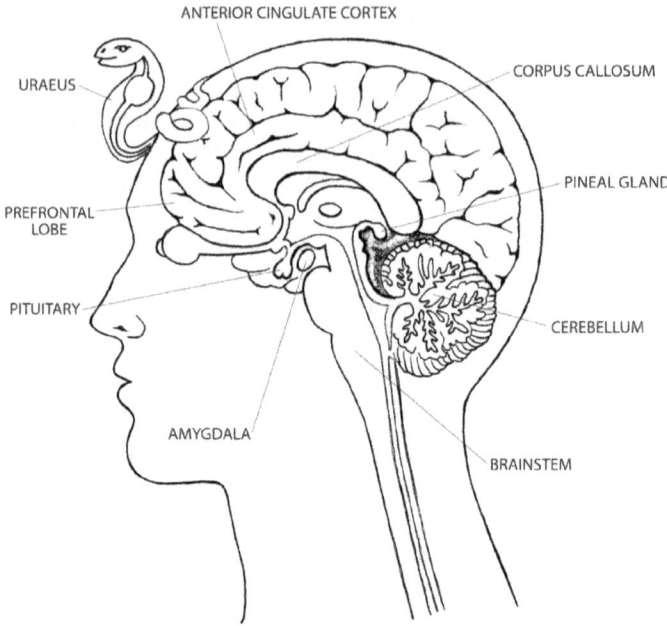

Sometimes when linking into the Uraeus in a semi-darkened room you can sense or see the capstone of the pyramid with the Eye of Horus within. That is by focusing on Uraeus you can see a white line tracing a triangle between the outer corners of the eyes and the apex of the forehead and in the middle you can see the Eye of Horus.

The Uraeus, for the purposes of sovereignty Inner Arts, is achieved via the unification of the subconscious, conscious and superconscious through removing dissonance, blocks and divisions. Coherence creates the ecstatic plasticity (surrender) necessary to come into sublime conjunction...ie: to download Spirit. It is this nexus I call the "cosmic umbilical" that gives us a sense of unification with the universe. Cosmic unification allows us to transcend all smallness, brokenness, disease, madness, poverty, deprivation, death, division, separation and alienation that constitutes the flatland world of the five senses.

The Muse comes through the right brain so to speak from the solar plexus and heart brains and their coherence with Zeropoint and the 8 Hz of Gaia. Then depending on the rational development and the technical skill, strength of character, vitality of body and power of will—the artistic creation is given birth into this world from Eternity and the ether. I theorize that one of the reasons why contact with the Muse rises to unbelievably Godlike proportions during a kundalini awakening is due to the extreme hyperactivation of the left-brain and left side of the body, which creates such an overload on those systems that the left-brain dominance is lifted and we begin to see and hear the world more through right-brain consciousness. At which point we see past the veil of the normal material domain to observe the poetic realm of archetype, psychic phenomena, visions, and gnostic revelation. Nature opens her vaults of secrets and infinity pours forth.

To focus on the Uraeus the eyeballs are turned up to the center of the forehead at the hairline. This is the throne of the sublime, beneficent presence within. It is interesting that no spiritual tradition other than the Egyptians has even hinted that this psychospacial region harbored the cosmic connection point. Because this knowledge must have been kept for the pharaohs and the Followers of Horus. However within the spiritual iconology and religious paintings you do see the eyes raised, and the One between the Two as familiar symbols. The Uraeus is the key to personal sovereignty, nobility, maturity and self-dominion.

Instead of clear disclosure of our spiritual hardware there is a serious distracting divergence occurring with people's preoccupation on the pineal gland. Leaving the eyes not raised high enough to draw the breath and build the ultimate plasma of Self. To establish the Uraeus eyeballs must be raised to a point about 3" out from the hairline, at which point an elongated triangle is formed — which is the same shape as the "Bread of the presence of God," Mfkzt or Shewbread. That is the tall pyramid shaped piles of monatomic white powder of gold mixed with frankincense and myrrh. The mana from Heaven (no place) is the Golden Tear from the Eye of Horus, achieved via sympathetic resonance between the crystalline body's EMF and the universe. The bindu point of the pyramid on which the Phoenix (bird of regeneration) alights is the apex the eyes point to when they focus on the head of the cobra of the Uraeus.

Our highest navigational coordinates originate from the seat of active compassion and active hope at the throne of Self-determination. The royal seat of Self is the Uraeus…the harmonizing governing point that synchronizes activity within and between the left and right hemispheres. Through this bird's eye vantage point we have the foresight to know right from wrong, and we automatically resolve the conflict between the self and the world. Having overcome our narcissism and the blindness of shadow we become a leader not only of our own lives, but are fit to lead others.

There is a dramatic increase in high-frequency brain activity called gamma waves during active compassion meditation. A gamma wave is a pattern of neural oscillation associated with attention and memory with a frequency between 25 to 100 Hz. The whole-brain integrating frequency (40 Hz) is typical in generating a mental state in which compassion permeates the whole mind with no other thoughts. Activity in the left prefrontal cortex (the seat of positive emotions such as happiness) acted to dominate or swamp activity in the right prefrontal (site of negative emotions and anxiety), thereby raising the synchronization of information processing within and between multiple brain areas.

Sublime connectivity with the infinite or universal Self gives us a bird's eye vantage point creating harmony between the self and the world, while the cooked culture creates the non-connectivity of the separate self sense. Because in the cooked food world we have generally created stagnant, acidic, toxic and hypoxic conditions in the body we are only accessing a fraction of our cognitive and spiritual abilities. Thus when we try and focus towards higher spin functioning it takes conscious effort to get enough oxygen into our system to reverse the acidic, toxic stagnation so we can "make contact" with our Self.

With more developed mastery over Prefrontal Lobe command, we are better able to modify and calm the limbic and reptilian brain which alters our entire metabolism, consciousness, behavior and experience because the Hypothalamus transforms the activity of the Prefrontal Lobes into hormonal messenger molecules. Both old brain and new brain meditative practices are essential to integrate and coordinate whole-brain functioning.

• URAEUS MEDITATION

The symbol of the Uraeus, or serpent's head at the top of the forehead, was used by the Egyptians as a royal symbol associated with transformation and evolution ie: sovereignty. This is the Bindu Point—the soul's pilot light, or the sovereign helm by which we reign ourselves into a coherent holy, whole. In my experience the Uraeus is at the hairline and is fed by a superluminal field of directed consciousness/energy. This is the focus point for maturity, for without coherency there is little depth, Presence, occupation, involvement, engagement or evolvement.

The focal point for the eyes in the Uraeus meditation is 3" or so in front of the hairline because the closed eyeballs have to laser together at a single point in combination with a fully opened throat, face and jaw in order to allow the heart and the anterior frontal lobes to resonate in sympathetic resonance. Thus this meditation requires the ongoing and progressive suspension and surrender of the egoic, analytic left brain and our personal narrative associated with our life's journey within Borg society. That is, in order to BUILD a brain for "transcendence" we cannot be invested in maintaining hold of our mundane and reactive self. Our mystical, magical and divine Self is always already a part of us. We have but to develop the neuro-circuitry to be able to access it in our daily life

Focusing the eyeballs directs consciousness and therefore conscious faculty, neurochemistry, neurogenesis and the quintessence or Presence. Focusing the eyeballs 3" in front of the hairline as in the Uraeus acts to produce the neurochemistry of maturity or "sovereignty." This is so because the anterior frontal lobes are the executive governing structure in the hierarchy of the brain. To the degree that we have not established superior communication with our inner pilot is the degree to which we are subject to domination, manipulation and seduction by other people, and blown about by happenstance and phenomena. We become intimate with our beneficent leader within by focusing the eyeballs on the Uraeus in meditation and drawing energy and breath into the area.

To do this we must build up our cellular energy, fluency of communication in the body, strength of the nerves, contact and resonance with Nature in order to generate a coherent laser focus on the presidential power of the soul. Furthermore we must have both the courage and the love to be willing to know our Self and become who we truly are.

All of the Inner Arts…the dropping of the muscles at the back of the tongue, the inner smile and the sensorially throaty breath. This is never more important than in the Uraeus meditation because without syncing the brain hemispheres, the on/off sides of the autonomic nervous system, and connecting the felt body to the head, you cannot create coherency between the heart and the executive brain. Although all the Inner Arts assist in some aspect of becoming fully HUman it is the Uraeus meditation that is the most incisive, penetrating and concentrated method for both palpating one's progress and facilitating sovereign mastery. For only we ourselves know how surrendered we are to our own heart, and how embodied we are in our own forehead.

By "Presence" I refer to the "felt-sense" of spiritual embodiment. It involves "dropping" into or melting into the full-sensory moment without resistance (push, pull, shove, retreat). Grace is when the body, mind and soul enter into sublime conversation. That is, the chariot, the horse and the driver are all going in the same direction without hesitation or debate. When inner-conjugation or love-making occurs from the quantum level right through to the Total Organism level then "I and the Father are One, we are the Christ, in cosmic consciousness, or we are sovereign.

The tongue is dropped into the belly to switch on the parasympathetic nervous system and the closed eyes are turned up towards the pilot seat at the hairline. This upward turn of the eyeballs focused on the apex is necessary to access the Uraeus-Heart connection that calms the bodymind's frequency toward maximum sympathetic resonance (coherence). It may be difficult at first to delve into these circuits as we are not used to energetically exploring this area of the brain and it is difficult to weld energy into this elevated point. When feeling into the regality of the Uraeus note that it emerges into a central point "beyond" the front of the cranium itself. You should feel electrical sensations coalescing into the quintessence of the cobra's head—the serpent of the Sun—at which point the separate-self-sense drops away.

The forward felt-sense of the brain, when you project the sense of prefrontal lobes out to a point 3" out from the hair line, is like a resonant connector point for upgrading the Anterior Cingulate Cortex. The ACC is like the roots to the Uraeus. It is useful to think of all forms in the body as being trees. You draw energy into the canopy of the tree while simultaneously feeding the roots, this makes a complete circuit or radiant EMF egg in each area you are working on. Remember radiance is synonymous with grounding and connection. Focusing consciousness at the Uraeus, into a cobra-like projection at the top of the forehead, is the quickest way to obliterate the negative vibration and distress from our interaction with the competitive world. One could call it the nondual, prima materia, primordial or diamond light that allows us the composure and coherence to shift our focus and become a ruler over our world.

Only intentional awareness or Presence allows for direct experience, otherwise we merely see through the lens of our own conditioning, projections, desires, fears and habits. Without consciousness converging through the upper anterior frontal lobes we do not rule our inner kingdom—that is we are not sovereign. The Fair Witness or transcendent consciousness is that dynamic magic that can spin gold from straw and allow us to travel through the valley of the shadow of death without being harmed. The irony is that we have to transcend the world in order to be fully Present in it! Horror, oblivion, and obliviousness seem to go together, this is what has gotten us into this predicament. If we are moving away from Reality we become progressively number and dumber.

Without unblocking the brain stem with the Core Supercharger, clearing out the emotional spindle cell network with the Heart-tree Meditation and building up the Uraeus we remain Pavlovian slaves to the dictates of outer forces and conditions, or pushed and pulled around by inner unconscious drives. Freud's superego is an inner uncertainty-absorbing device, an interiorized boss. This "friendly boss" resides at the Uraeus, the cohesive leader of the integrated brain that binds together the assertive and nurturing instincts—thus synergizing self, other and We.

Through neuronal development we can grow our boss to become beneficent, secure, egalitarian, nurturing, affirming, and cooperative AS WELL AS assertive, decisive, agentic, creative, enterprising, and materially successful. Thus we marry the best of the masculine and feminine within the focal bindu point of the sovereign's will power…the Uraeus. The Phoenix of the soul alights on the Bindu, which is why the winged serpent and the sun are perhaps the most common motifs of spiritual iconography. Use the Thymus Light Sword and the Uraeus Meditation in the same meditation for powerfully synergistic effects.

To set your inner child free to create, you have to elect yourself the beneficent ruler of your own inner kingdom, in order to overcome the brain retarding influence of automatic unconscious fear generated sadomasochistic socio-emotional programming. The most succinct method of doing this is connecting the heart to the Uraeus (prefrontal lobes). By doing the heart-Uraeus meditation the anterior frontal lobes and the heart click into sympathetic resonance…the more effective we are at this meditation the more we embody spiritual maturity, mastery and the Muse, for we have established higher executive control over the runaway programs of our social animal heritage.

Meditation has been associated with decreased stress, depression, anxiety, pain and insomnia, and an increased quality of life. Meditation actually increases the thickness of the cortex in areas involved in attention and sensory processing, such as the prefrontal cortex and the right anterior insula. This growth of the cortex is not due to the growth of new neurons, but results from wider blood vessels, more supporting structures such as glia and astrocytes, and increased dendrite branching and connections.

We cannot change others, but we CAN change the way we respond to them.

THE KABALA AND THE EGG

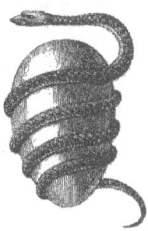

I interpret chakras or Sephiroth as the metaphysical Spiral Dynamics chart of the levels of consciousness placed in the body, but their linear aspect is deceiving. Actually the line of ascendancy is circular in that the Uroboros really must bite its tail, or the wholism of consciousness is "broken." To the extent that the higher fails to marry or communicate with the lower, is the extent to which the organism is obsolete and in oblivion. Thus our crown chakra is as "opened" or healthy (whole) as our base chakra is opened, or healthy (whole). Kundalini doesn't necessarily start anywhere because it is a whole-system alchemy — so all parts of you from zeropoint, subatomic to your galactic self are the "origins" or the cause of kundalini.

The reason why the upper and lower are One is that the EMF of the body is an egg, so the upper means nothing without the lower and the lower means nothing without the upper. The egg and Uroboros are refracted holographically throughout all of creation on all levels. This is the first principle of fractality we should be taught in kindergarten, but most of us never learn it at all, which is why we have a neurotic, anxious and schizophrenic society slavishly conforming to social roles and stereotypes.

If the base chakra is dead, then so too will be the crown chakra, in fact the crown will literally feel numb if the pelvic plexus is atrophied. Life and authenticity demand that we overcome our resistance to incorporating the base and crown chakras. The force of Kundalini will undertake to unite all parts of our being in one luminous whole. Thus, our psychic exercises, and esoteric meditations are designed to prepare our minds, bodies, and consciousness for the liberation of the Sacred Fire of the Void. Buried in matter, is a underlying vibrant energy that is continually pulsating, giving rise to form and life, and turning energy in matter and matter into energy.

Through a progressive shedding, detoxification, cleansing of the body, the fire of consciousness is liberated, allowing the ever present power and energy, of spirit to be released. Thus, the divine power of the serpent doesn't really sleep, it is we who are asleep to its presence and unestimatible blessing. To be sovereign is to be free of conditioned habit and the coercive control of others — to truly direct our own life. The throne room, or seat of sovereignty is the crystal palace, that is the.pineal-pituitary chamber, while the helm is the Uraeus. The whole brain integrating Gamma Frequency 40Hz is accessed through prefrontal ignition by raising the eyeballs into the Upper forehead in the Uraeus meditation, but the body must be released of its stress for whole brain syncopation to occur. Thus doing strenuous lower lung breathing, using the upper stomach muscles to push the diaphragm in on the out-breath allows the body to relax enough for whole brain harmonization. Deep breathing in negative ions promotes alpha brainwaves and increases brainwave amplitude, which translates to a higher awareness level. Negative-ion induced alpha waves spread from the occipital area to the parietal and temporal and even reach the frontal lobes, spreading evenly across the right and left brain hemispheres.

Circulation of the Light, or the purification and strengthening of the Vital Energy through the Middle Pillar by grounding, imagination, breath, and concentration is the alchemical creation of the Philosopher's Stone giving one the ability to direct this Cosmic creative energy at will. This can be done by imagining your feet are rooted into the center of the earth, and energy can be felt running up the legs, as a pulse, entering the spinal column, and energizing the whole body as it pours out the top of the head — thus uniting heaven and earth.

It is apparent that we have enough physical abundance on the planet although badly distributed. We have enough mental/feeling abundance although badly integrated. What we are ailing for is a lack of genuine spiritual abundance. The "Tree of Life" offers a symbolic working model of creation on both the microcosmic and macrocosmic scales, in that the branches are nothing without the roots. It is time we fed the spiritual roots of the human tree for they are hungry for nutritious organic fertilizer. Through reaching for the stars within we will bring down the mana from the heavens to feed the entire human cosmos and the planet. What we need is a genuine nonsecular spirituality for the masses. A transformation in the trenches. It is time to bring the lotus of human potential into being.

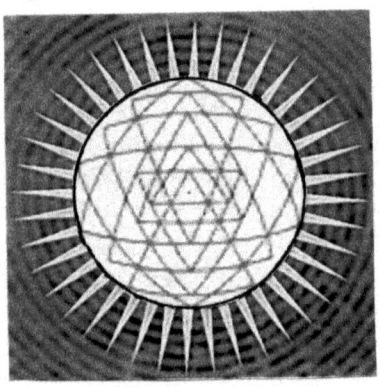

"We poor humans are taught from the beginning that our every act must have some sort of rational or moral purpose; that our actions must be "right." To justify what we do, we frequency require that others be wrong. The result is endless unnecessary conflict." ~ Luke Rhinehart, The Book of the Die.

CHAPTER 4

PRINCIPLE SOVEREIGNTY PRACTICES

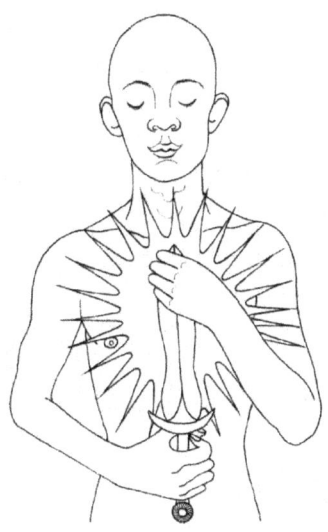

• LIGHT SWORD MEDITATION

(*Thymus Gland Illumination*) Regular practice of the thymus light sword meditation will promote socioemotional and physical immunity "without the effort of mind or muscle," and increase your sense of integrated wholeness, as well as improving the intelligence of the immune system. The sword is made of light and laid on the chest, with the tip of the blade just above the clavicle, and the hilt of the sword held below the sternum. Put one hand at the clavicle and the other at the solar plexus as though holding the tip and the hilt of a short sword. Feel Excalibur deep inside the sternum and get the sense that the sword is radiating with light. Feel the thymus gland become warm as it begins to vibrate and expand like a radiant sun; keep the vibrancy of the sword alive by breathing deeply with a throaty breath. The throaty breath acts like a bellows on the generation and radiation of light.

The Light Sword gives you a focused presence in the central command center of your immune system, and a powerful shield for your heart. This position allows you to collect your energies and focus on building the immune system in one powerful pose. You may feel areas lacking in Life Force such as a breast, liver, spleen or at the back of the heart. Focus the mind's eye on these deprived or wounded areas and send breath, Life Force and light into their pain or emptiness. A LED Light Crystal Wand can also be held over the thymus gland on the chest as a "real" light sword.

• LIGHT SWORD AND URAEUS MEDITATION COMBO

The light sword and the Uraeus are the vehicle of discernment whereby all else is dropped in order to quantum cohere to the majestic core of being. When we build up the thymus (CIA) of the immune system's superconducting communications and open the Stargate to infinity (The Uraeus) at the center of the prefrontal cortex, we no longer have to use our emotions, muscles or will to defend ourselves from attack, interference, loss, shattering or deconstructive forces. Rather than putting our precious energy into defense – which automatically invites attack – we are better off merely claiming the apriori strength and nobility that is already ours.

Once we embody our majesty through connection to Source, we can no longer be under-mined and made less than we are…we become the new nobility…The Titans. The paradox is that if we defend against an apparent enemy we become them. For then we get lost in their reality bubble rather than focusing directly on proactively realizing our own potential, without the need to fight off that which we deem counter to our weal-being (whole-integrated self). That is we cannot unify and come into quantum coherence when in resistance to any part of it. (Which provides the counter logic to the idea of holy war).

The more we awaken to the light, the deeper into the shadows we can see.

• BLUE SPOT MEDITATION

The Blue Spot (*Locus coeruleus*) is the noradrenalin spark plug for alertness, awareness and Presence. The goal of presence practices is to prevent our emotional affect running away so we can gain greater stabilization of our autonomic nervous system, whereby we conserve energy and raise oherency for neurogenesis and initiation of the mature sovereign, self-dominion or self-possession. Without raw tissues, Omega-3, remineralization, grounding and sunlight, combined with high quality structured water we fail to produce optimum cellular hydration and metabolism. Any deviation away from optimal conditions for Life is a step towards death.

This meditative exercise is for charging the entire nervous system with electrons and photons to reduce inflammation, and the hyperactivation of the sympathetic nervous system. It incorporates the synergistic effects of grounding, solar photons, breathing and full body integrative focus. In the nude or in thin natural fabric, lie on the ground with your exposed feet facing the sun. This meditation is good to do under a tree with the head facing the trunk. Ideally the ground should be slightly damp to facilitate electron flow. If there are creepy crawlies about then put down a large cotton sheet to lie on. Put two fingers in the Mouth of God at the apex of the spine and press down on the forehead at the Third Eye with two fingers of the other hand to increase pressure. Focus on the Mind's Eye, which is the "felt-sense connection" between these two points. After you have centered and connected yourself you can drop the hand at your forehead to your solar plexus.

Do the Inner Smile, drop the muscles at the back of the tongue, and Hum inside your head occasionally to keep your Mind's Eye more awake. The inner smile lights up the Blue Spot with indigenous satiety. Once you have established the connection of the Mind's Eye on the Blue Spot (or the back of the brainstem), then breathe in through the top of your head and send this awareness-charge down the body to the feet with each out breath—feeling the breath mate with the sun's rays on your feet! The brain communicates with your toes within a few thousandths of a second. The coccygeal gland in the sacrum may start pulsating and you should feel the splay of pelvic nerves feeding on the ground energy and will experience more energy and sensation radiating down the legs. As the body absorbs energy the diaphragm will relax, breathing will normalize and the cells will get more oxygen and become less acidic. With the electrons from the ground the red blood cells clump less, carry more oxygen and blood and lymph is less "sticky" when it is properly charged with negative ions from the ground.

After a while turn over and allow your front side to feed on the ground energy and your back to feed on the sun. Place your jaw directly on the grass for grounding, and put two fingers in the Mouth of God with the other hand. Turn your eyeballs up to your crown and breath in through your feet and with the out-breath pull the charge up your body and out the top of your head. Toning is particularly good while on your stomach because you can really feel the resonance in your head and it allows you to extend the breath longer than you otherwise would. Continue the Blue Spot meditation for half an hour each side, (especially if you don't do it everyday), as it takes a while for the body to feed on the negative ions from the ground and the positive charge (voltage) of the Sun's rays.

The Blue Spot meditation is the primo ultra sovereignty exercise for very rapid neuro-restructuring, integration and rebalancing. The background information on this is extensive and focuses on melanin and the locus coeruleus (Blue Spot) as the noradrenalin spark plugs of the sympathetic arousal system. The Blue Spot meditation shifts the body out of chronic hyperarousal, because it is being fed the energy it needs to overcome inflammation and free radical oxidation and for normalizing cellular chemoelectrical, pH and osmotic gradients. With the Blue Spot Meditation we provide the ions for the zeta-potential, energy and the information integration for the holistic unification of bodymind and soul.

The Blue Spot Meditation lays the cellular groundwork for establishing immunity from internal defensive triggers and social pathology. by hyper-integrating the bodymind. We cannot willingly engage in the old systems of behavior, thought and conversation without denying, betraying and negating our Self. As we reconnect and inner commune we repair our neuroemotional system and establish community in which "sovereign sensitivity" is the bottom-line. Through learning to calm ourselves down to maintain our cosmic connection we stabilize our sense of sovereign dignity and non-separation.

It is important to do Inner Arts in nature to normalize the spectrum of the energy frequencies and to amplify the feeling of cosmic connection (soul-amplification).

• MITOCHONDRIA MEDITATION

"I was in an hour long Mitochondria Meditation session. I had non-stop jumps. I am so excited with my initial contact. In my session, I was completely naked and I was floating in the Universe. I felt the beauty of my body. I felt the breeze, the moon light, I landed on the moon and fooled around with rocks and looked down at the earth. When I visualized the cells and sent lights to the mitochondria, all the body/mind armor are disintegrated. I no longer need the usual stuff to protect me! I Am at the quantum level, I Am one with the Universe. The prohibition of Eros is being blasted away by my lighted mitochondria.

During my mitochondria meditation with hands and feet connected last night, as soon as I sent light to my core mitochondria, my hands felt numb, then they started to beat with a distinct rhythm. The palms and all the fingers were beating with a pattern. The beating soon synced up with the beating of my brainstem. My hands were heavy and magnetic as if they are drawing blood/prana from my body. I had to get up at 4am to walk because the energy was busting me out of bed... Now I know there is an infinite supply of energy within us..." ~ Debbie M

The Mitochondria Meditation is the alpha and omega of sovereignty practice, with the other Inner Arts being training ground for this deepest permission, liberation and motivation of the soul. The Mito Meditation is for directly touching of the Sacred Feminine and uplink to the Goddess, the Creatrix, Sophia and Gaia. Because the mitochondria are the source of energy generation they are the source of consciousness. With this meditation we use consciousness to touch consciousness and thereby facilitate dynamic metamorphosis, using deeply penetrating awareness to build up the neurological and biochemical richness of the inner HUman.

To transcend the hardening of surface Borgman we must love ourself more than the world can love us. But we must go beyond an intellectual understanding of loving ourselves and we cannot merely spout affirmations about self-love in the hope that it will sink in and be true. No, we must turn the light of our felt-awareness back on itself in unconditional love, appreciation and gratitude, as though falling in love with the cosmos from the inside out. In this way we "become" love and can love the world unconditionally, and so not be undone and hardened by it.

Sit in the easy chair position with a bolster under your knees (or in bed). Left hand on the heart, right hand on the solar plexus. Drop the muscles at the back of your tongue and do the Inner Smile, engage slow gentle deep belly breathing. Get the sense you are floating weightless and pull your minds eye into your inner core. Now sense the 100 trillion cells making up your body and feel into the mitochondria within the cells. Direct gratitude and love, a deep gentle, sweetness, welcoming encouragement and unconditional blessing (*beneficence*) into your mitochondria...thanking them for producing the fuel that fires up your existence and lights the way.

The more you direct your focus into your energy producing plants the greater they will come forth in response, to produce more energy, more clarity and greater efficiency...thereby undoing stress, dysfunction and aging at its source. The highest instrument of consciousness (the frontal lobes) becomes a flood lamp that shines loving acknowledgement on the energy generating plants in our starship body. The Uroboros of the beginning and ending Grok in infinite embrace. Through gratitude we raise the generation of cellular energy (ATP) such that communication/communion becomes perfect, or non-separate, that is non-local. This means short wavelength = high frequency = more energy, long wavelength = low frequency = less energy.

That which is actively loved grows stronger…this is the mothering energy that "derepresses" suspended epigenetic expression. The fundamental axiom of Life is that it is environment created and creates environment. We can love ourselves into incarnating a greater degree of Self by the quality of attention we give to our cells. You have to be unconditionally happy and bliss-filled to make healthy love to your mitochondria and in return, they will take you to the moon and back. Turning the light around to appreciate the organelle that drives our spaceship is the flip of the switch into hyperdrive. If the body is a starship, the mitochondrion is its engine room. When you tune into your engine room with conscious loving intent and gratitude (especially first thing in the morning before rising from bed) you green light yourself and liberate your energy stores for the day. This self-loving attention is contagious, and so others imbibe self-care and empowerment from our switched on self-loving bodymind.

It is interesting that if you have discombobulated your nervous system with stress (cortisol) or food that is exhausting for the body to process it is very hard to focus on the mitochondria. The inflamed, incoherent body also can't conjure up gratitude, because the liver is overtaxed, and gratitude is a very highly cohesive, conjugated frequency. This points to the need for a stress reduction and clean-living lifestyle in order to manifest maximum ATP/light. We need high ATP levels and coherent light to generate Gamma wave frequency in the prefrontal lobes. It takes the supreme focus of Gamma wave to "touch" the mitochondria with love, hence liberate the focused attention needed for learning and memory. We literally re-member our Self through focusing the light of our loving attention inward.

Remember the mitochondria hold a different set of genes based on the female line of descent, so by green lighting them, you support the epigenetic expression of genes which may have been repressed/depressed during the struggle of females within the competitive, oppositional and anti-Eros culture. During Mitochondrial Meditation you can feel more activity in the right side of the brain, thus we can lift the lid placed on our feminine intelligence (intuition, empathy, synthesis, wholism, Psi, visions, gnosis). By freeing feminine receptive energy from the shaming of Eve and fully showing up as a force of sanity, balance and felt-presence we can pull the human race back from the brink of destruction.

The Inner Arts are the principle form of bonding whereby we attain a deeper relationship with our Self and hence a deeper relationship with the cosmos. By establishing this primary connection we are less likely to be pulled off track into unhealthy entropic relationships that dis-integrate our integrity and waste our time and energy. The more we establish an integrative Uraeus (Gamma wave) meditative connection to our mitochondria, the more we build our sovereign core. In the beginning this communication/communion with your mitochondria is definitely an "exercise," and as you gain success with the meditative contact, you can feel the body do a jump or jolt, like moving through threshold levels of self-recognition or self-remembering.

Initially self-love takes an enormous concentration to establish dynamic Presence, but results are immediate. As well as sending gratitude to your mitochondria spend some time sending gratitude to your liver as well, for the colossal processing service it does for you. Send gratitude to any other part of the body that is troubling you to bring it back into the wholeness of the integrated starship. The powering up of the Merkaba lightship is achieved through the gamma wave connection with the mitochondria. Link the gamma wave Uraeus with the proton vectors of the mitochondrial membranes and we materialize through stargates to greater incarnation in this dimension by jumping to higher octaves in energy valence—to generate the heroic state.

The Mito Meditation focus of gratitude toward the mitochondria is one of the best methods of installing abundance programming of the cells. Because abundance comes from appreciation for that which we already have. There must be apriori fullness and satisfaction in order to rise out of deprivation consciousness, poverty, fight/flight and criminal gain. Abundance is "built" by rising beyond neediness and raising the body's energy and frequency to the radiant-giving level, through which gnosis, genius, synchronicity, enterprise, adventure, true fun and joy can occur. Once we are in "right HUman relationship" to the universe — abundance just falls into play from the coordinating resonant energy of our own cellular gratitude and appreciation—radiance and depth.Mito Meditation is best done first thing in the morning prior to the mask of the daily personality descending, which locks us into a habitual level of energy/consciousness associated with our past conditioning.

• LYMPHATIC BREATHING

Stagnation of lymphatic function in the thoracic duct supraclavicular lymph nodes is associated with insufficient belly breathing due to stress, trauma and PTSD. This backing up of lymph causes ongoing physiological dysregulation, brain fog and disorientation. Conscious lymphatic breathing is a fundamental vote for our own wellbeing and increases the body's voltage so that damaged tissue regenerates, and internal organs come back to vital life! Sit or lie in the sun and sungaze with eyes open or closed depending on the sun's height in the sky. Do deep breathing and pull the stomach muscles into the diaphragm on the huffy out-breath to stimulate and move the lymph nodes that run along the thoracic lymphatic tract between the belly button and the chest. Huuing or humming will add vibratory stimulation to help clear the lymphatic system. Use lymphatic breathing for the following exercise and other Inner Arts. It is powerful if done in the bath, or in bed first thing in the morning while still in bed. Put a shungite disc on your Thymus (sternum) during the lymphatic breathing to amplify the effects.

Harmony and balance can be established with the Core SuperCharger.

• THE CORE SUPERCHARGER

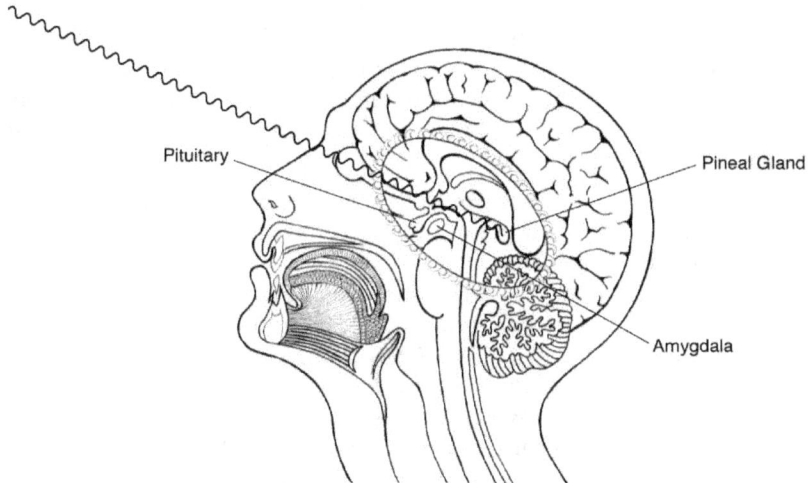

The Core SuperCharger, or brain-sex, is the principle alchemical sovereignty exercise for clearing, charging and integrating the whole brain. It calms, cleans and makes receptive (ascends) the lower brain structures so that they are more pliant to the influence of the Prefrontal Lobes (Uraeus). The top of the brainstem is like a penis inside a vagina, against the cervix and womb. Thus the crystal chamber is an alchemical vessel for the generation of charged bioplasma, which ionizes cerebrospinal fluid and clears blockage on all scales. The most intense work we must do at the beginning stages of awakening sovereignty is to clean out the brainstem bringing body, mind and intention into a seamless focused flow. Thus brain-sex is quintessential alchemy as it is truly evolutionary.

The Core SuperCharger is undeniably brain sex, whereas The Pot of Gold is pure relaxed ecstasy. Self in-to-me-see or coming back to our Self for the first time is both shocking and laced with a sense of grief for having been parted with ourselves for so long. Sit-lie relaxed in an easy chair posture with knees raised, the head supported and eyes closed and turned toward natural light or a candle. Felt-sense an Inner Smile with ears raised. The body of the tongue is raised towards the palate, while the back of the tongue muscles are relaxed. You can do the core supercharger without sunlight on the eyelids, but it is not as effective at generating the plasma ball.

With the eyes closed look back down through your optic nerves at the glowing ball of plasma in the cup of your jaw that is created by the felt-sense of the Inner Smile. While doing this charge the plasma fire ball with oxygen by using the nose as a bellows to pull large breaths into the brain-core. Breathing into the masterful seat of the womb of the brain expedites the process. The location of the pineal gland is near the upper end of the spinal cord, which ends or terminates in the oldest anatomical region in the brain…the crystal chamber.

The backward flip of the mind's eye into the core of the brain, in combination with light, oxygen and attention produces a harmonizing fusion between the pineal (male) and pituitary (female) glands in the crystal chamber. This repolarizes, resets and recharges the cerebellum and brainstem, and soothes the hypothalamus and the amygdala. Healing the brain-core liberates the prefrontal lobes to engage their executive organizing more efficiently. If done for 15-30 minutes this charges, lightens, revitalizes, integrates the whole body and it builds indomitable Presence.

When the jaw is in the Inner Smile this produces significant bliss, thus providing a container for the difficult process of looking backwards through the optic nerves. The Core Supercharger takes "turning the light around" literally. When you succeed in turning the focus down you will see a warm glow of orange light. Thus if you have sunlight photons hitting your eyeballs you can easily imagine the light feeding the inner alchemy in the central cauldron of the brain. By looking down the optic nerves the eyeballs are turned down in their sockets, which exposes more of the top of the eyeball towards the solar light. Solar influence comes through the receptors in the top of the eye (not through the seeing part). Even with the eyelids closed this allows more of a direct flow of solar-subtle energy down into the pituitary area which then feeds the pineal gland. The Sun stands universally for the supramental Light, the divine Gnosis."

You might run into a problem if you do too much core supercharging without adequate grounding. It is amazing how fast the core supercharger meditation ephemeralizes, refines energy and quickens consciousness. By focusing on the brain core in this way we pay quality attention to our deep self and fill ourselves up with nectar. The pineal gland has direct relationship to the sun. René Descartes called the pineal gland the point of interaction between the spirit and body. He regarded it as the principal seat of the soul and the place in which all our thoughts are formed.

• BASE CORE SUPERCHARGER

Because it heals on such a core level the Core Supercharger simultaneously lights up the plasma charge in the area between the perineum and the Hara. Just like you focus on the plasma ball in the "dish" of the jaw, you can then shift your focus down to this spot just above the pubic bone and build significant ambrosial plasma ball there. Women can also put the mind's eye on the G-spot while doing Kegel's contractions and conscious breathing. In the male body the sweet spot for focus the mind's eye is the male G spot, which located inside midway between the scrotum and the anus. You need character strength to do this and not sexualize the bliss energy into egoic masturbatory stimulation. We must drop our ego addiction in order to truly love ourselves and overcome our fear of sovereignty. The challenge to the ego-personality is to not "masturbate" and waste the charge, because the sovereign light body needs all the energy it can get from the pupal body in order to transmute and restructure it. I doubt anyone can become sovereign without this exercise or something similar such as Taoist energy cultivation.

The dish of the jaw correlates to the dish of the pelvic bone. The brain plasma ball and the base plasma ball are like the north and south pole—they are two halves of the same thing that "co-arise." Having the knees bent frees up energy flow in the pelvic area so the two poles of the charge can conjunct. Uni-polar ascension (primary dualism) is obviously a false bias of the "specialness" of the ego. The two poles automatically arise during charging to advance from disjunction to conjunction The many become one, the components participating equally in the concrescence. Everything finally comes together in a harmonious nexus of completion, orgasm or unity—connecting to the core or the center.

• EMPOWERING THE BRAINSTEM

To build power in the brainstem press two fingers in the notch near the Foramen Magnum, the dip where the spine goes into the skull. Turn your eyeballs down to look back at the area of the brainstem where your fingers are and focus energy and attention there. The Mind's Eye just naturally goes to the "sweet spot," which is an area around the pituitary gland at the top of the brainstem. Feel the presence of apriori unconditional health and power in the brainstem while repeating such words as power, presence, health, focus, peace, strength, and glory in this area. This can be done while lying on your back, sitting or riding a bus and if you do it while looking the sun with your eyelids closed you can use the photons to catalyze the meditation. You will probably find after ten minutes or so, that you can feel a strong center of bliss-plasma in the brainstem, which is often the sorest, numb spot on the body. Luminous ambrosia or liquid light radiates from the brainstem, filling your body, clarifying and cleansing any problem, dissonance or separation.

A blissful ball of atomic plasma builds in the brainstem, which may be difficult to integrate if you do not breathe into the pressure, as though giving birth to yourself. There are plentiful opiate endorphin, cannaboid and GABA receptors in the brainstem, which we are not normally aware of without directed meditation. Bliss is the result of the building and charging of coherent biophoton flow…essentially "opening" latent poorly accessed neuron capacity and strengthening consciousness (Presence). Charged bodies that are more highly organized are going to obviously perform better and deeper as complex instruments of multplexival consciousness. Full cellular energy (kundalini) is needed for connection, communication, communion, without which there is no phase conjugation, or inner-conjunction.

"All motion is as omnipresent as the Light of God is omnipresent. All effect is universal. God is balance. From the stillness of His balance in the unconditioned One Light, He extends His balance to the conditioned universe of motion as two opposite unbalanced conditions of two lights, which seek balance through each other. Equal interchange between opposite conditions manifests the love principle of balance upon which God's universal body is founded." ~ Walter Russell, p.76 The Divine Iliad, vol.1

• CONEHEAD MEDITATION

I have been contemplating the neuro-acoustical properties of the shape of the "conehead" and that this has immediate mind-substance altering effects! It is easy to change the energy flow and resonance in the skull by felt-sensing oneself to have a conehead. The muscles at the back of the ears cock-up when doing this and breathing naturally deepens due to the increased oxygen demands of heightened consciousness. The Conehead meditation helps repair the primary vehicle of the EMF egg - uniting top and bottom as One. You can feel an instant nobility, majesty, presence, purpose and power in merely sensing your head as though it was that of a conehead. For this meditation, sit in a comfy chair with one knee bent up so you can prop up your elbow and rub the fontanel spot on the top of your head.

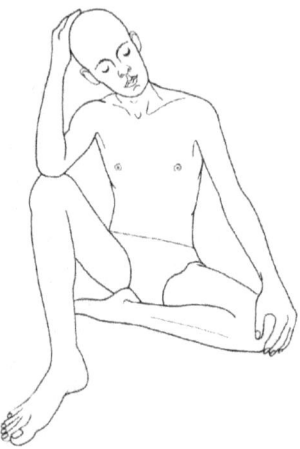

Sitting semi-upright on a chair with both legs on the seat, you will probably be using your right hand to rub, but you can use the knee of either leg to prop your arm up to your head. The top of the crown may feel dense and numb, as though unawakened. Do the Inner Smile and extend it back and up through the cerebellum, right up to the crown. So now, with the Inner Smile running up the back of the skull to the top of the head, and the knee cocked up to allow the crown to be rubbed without effort — begin humming Huuuu with mouth closed to allow a full resonant vibration to be felt throughout the skull and sensed by the fingertips as they rub the fontanel in circular motion.

The sense of connection, non-separation, unity, wholeness and presence is the sovereign thrival state. This amplified communication/communion or intimacy with the soul is a consequence of the biological faith that results from high cell voltage, and fast-speed connection to the cosmos. This is a raw, alkaline, high electron donor (reducing) antioxidant state with a marked absence of toxins and blockage on all scales from subatomics to thought processes. We naturally want to be respectful, reverential and in awe, because these are significantly high-energy states of "connection," however there is not a whole lot in our daily lives that stimulates mystical wonder and humility and gratitude. For now, the coneheads provide us with a mind-expanding dose of respect, reverence and bewilderment. It is very important to reconstitute the crown area of the brain which is the seat of awakeness vs. narcosis and retardation.

• CROWN CHAKRA MEDITATION

Any genius taps into the trans-normal, whether they admit to the transpersonal realm is just a matter of how "secure" their ego is. The seventh seal or crown chakra must be opened to loosen the self-repressive and separative instincts of the defensive ego that renders us unconscious (nescience). The crown chakra located at the crown of the head is your place of grokking, bliss, and divinity. The associated color is violet. When it is clear and open, it is our own personal vortical Stargate, or wormhole, into the higher dimensions. A harmonious Crown Chakra would mean a steady connection to transpersonal realm of Infinite Consciousness, as well as awareness and expression of the Unified Nature of Reality. It assists in receiving higher awareness for fulfilling our sovereign path and soul-purpose. By giving this Chakra love and attention, blockages are cleared, energy flow increases and the chakras are subsequentially balanced and healed in the process.

The crown chakra is ruled by the pineal gland and the melatonin spiritual chemistry cascade. Opening the crown chakra allows us to access our deep sleep (Delta) brainwaves while we are still somewhat awake. Thus through interpenetration of the levels of consciousness we access multidimensional and extrasensory senses and information. Once this chakra is opened, our sense of empathy and unity consciousness expands. We come home to feel "secure," united between Father Sky and Mother Earth.

With your eyelids closed turn your eyes upwards such that you are trying to see the ceiling or sky right through the top of your head. Do long slow deep breathing and feel every inhalation saturating the top of the head with blood, energy and light. Chant the sound *Nggg* or *Hmm*. The ability to perceive our physical life from that higher perspective of the Eye of Horus allows us to gain access to our multidimensional consciousness. Through connection, communication, and deep understanding of our higher-dimensional self we can remember the innate power and potential gifts that we were born with.

• OPENING THE BASE CHAKRA

Unplugging the brainstem and limbic system with the Core Supercharger works to open up the base chakra. Otherwise nude sunbathing on the genitals, alternating hot and cold, hot rocks, lying-sitting-meditating on the earth. Sunlight imparts charge and increases the viscosity of water so all work in the body is catalyzed and metabolism/detoxification is more efficient. Topical Syrian rue oil keys you into 8Hz, or the Schumann resonance of the planet opens the base chakra such that it is like floating on a magic carpet. Anything that kick starts the kundalini gland at the base of the spine will assist opening the base chakra. Traditionally yogis use bandhas (muscle contraction), pranayama (breathing), asanas (postures), tantra, meditation and visualization.

Meditating and sungazing at dawn and dusk while sitting on iron rich rocks greatly speeds up ascension. Fasting and colonics is perhaps one of the most effective means of unblocking energy flow as it gets rid of interference and stagnation right down to the atomic level. Vibratory machines, percussion massage tools and rebounder trampolines will also help to remove morbid material and energy and raise sentience and allow the energy to flow through the area activating the dormant potential of spirit embodiment by overcoming the rigidity of chronic spiritual disconnection. Once unblocked and activated more "light" can flow through the central channel of the spine (*sushumna*).

• THE POT OF GOLD

This culminating Inner Art turns off the sympathetic activation and removes worry, mental chatter and generates Presence and strengthens and tunes the parasympathetic nervous system, setting a blissful equanimous vibe prior to making decisions. Not only can Pot of Gold be used to alleviate depression it can also be used to enhance creativity. The **Amrita** chemicals produced in the brain during this process increase visual acuity and transcendental vision and Gnostic dream states. This is a simple method of generating ecstasy, peace and equanimity. You lie on your back on the floor or bed, put the left hand on the middle of the chest and the right hand on the solar plexus. Turn your head to the right, drop the tongue down into the belly, do the Inner Smile, focus the mind's eye on the brainstem and silently repeat the word "peace" with your gentle belly breathing. You can tone also, but beginners may find this extra element hard to include with so much to focus consciousness on. The more you generate a huge charge of peace-ecstasy with this technique the more you change your nervous system away from sympathetic activation of defense circuits, which generate nerve-static and high blood pressure.

• THE COSMIC WOMB

The **Shekinah** or feminine face of the godhead is the Cosmic Womb, the Palace, the Fountain, and Mystical Garden. Reprogramming limbic imprints helps us overcome repetitive negative emotions, as these produce helplessness and incoherence. To heal the broken inner child we must remarry the cosmic parents of earth and sky within our heart. In committed long term love relationship dopamine is stimulated for motivation and ongoing bonding… this provides the ideal conditions for the substantial gestation of a child. We can reprogram our initial deprivation wiring through the simulation of an ideal womb experience, thereby strengthening the heart-field to allow a cosmic sense of safety and self-recognition…in which higher sovereign neuro-circuitry can form.

Put on some soft evocative music and create a comfortable nest of cushions in the sun, lie in fetal position with sunlight on your face, do cleansing breaths and generate the Inner Smile. Build a plasma ball in the dish of the jaw by looking down through the back of your eyes. Visualize yourself in a sacred space in nature and imagine being in the belly of your Cosmic Mother with your Cosmic Father at her side. See your ideal soul parents interacting in fullness, wholeness and abundance expressing their undying love for each other.

This changes the fundamental socio-neural patterns within, normally unreachable by any other means than a true love relationship. The reconcillation of the inner parents allows you to draw on the nectar of the sanctuary of the Self on the deepest of levels. The Inner Marriage and "floating in the amniotic fluid of the cosmic womb "experience is vitally important to lay the foundation for reprogramming on higher levels. You have to "let go" of who you are to become who you will be. You may find that it gives a sense of warmth, fullness, sweetness and satiety to the inner "autonomic" brain regions. It also provides one with the sense of self-reliance, in that we can tend to our own core and are not dependent on anyone else for a sense of worthiness, well-being and surity. It is Ground Zero for emotional uplift and creative backbone.

• CEREBRAL UROBOROS MEDITATION

This important sovereignty exercise builds consciousness plasma-power in the brainstem, which is the "seat" of the Prefrontal Lobes. In this way we can directly "remother" ourselves into improved self-regulation and enhanced autonomic function…and through this remothering we can upgrade our Will to Live and get in touch with "Knowing Thyself." Healing the mother wound is central to our freedom and evolution as it is the Mother than gives us our original self-concept, and the ability to love ourselves inside our flesh on the atomic level every moment of our life.

For those who have suffered early trauma it is the brainstem that needs to be cleared and rewired in order to get more efficient flow into the rest of the brain and thus allow consciousness to become fully integrated. You will consciously have to "touch" whatever is numbing and separating you from unification as you work through the armor blockage in the brainstem. On working through resistance you acknowledge the negative-emotion, but you quickly replace it with gratitude, unity, awe, bliss or peace. For the longer you indulge in the maladative coping emotions the stronger their hold over you, and/or the more of your life wasted to anti-life, or that which is opposed to or restricting the full development of life.

The frontal lobes are connected via the reticulofrontal pathway from the front of the brainstem, which is responsible for arousal and activation. This allows conscious or executive control over the reptilian part of the brain that encompasses the brainstem, limbic system, and thalamus. It is this "unconscious part" that controls and runs all the automatic functions of the body which we are largely unaware of, allowing us to interact with our reality in a 'spontaneous' way. Thus the frontal lobe decision-making functions rely on the energy battery in the brainstem through the loop of the ascending mesocortical dopamine pathway. The mesocortical dopaminergic system exerts an inhibitory influence on the spontaneous activity or excitatory response induced from the main thalamic afferent on the prefrontal cortical cells.

Prefrontal decision-making thus comes full circle through a dopamine driven loop to our motion and motivation faculties...supporting our drives, the will to live, our agency and efficacy. The efficiency and complexity of our executive functions and personality thus relies on the healthy function of the brainstem and the smooth running of our autonomic functions. Also the prefrontal lobes succumb to the effects of aging more rapidly than the rest of the brain...and thus the myelin coating of the long interconnecting pathways of the brain is important to maintaining a youthful brain.

Dopaminergic insufficiency is the earliest and most severe disturbance of neuro-transmission accompanying the aging brain. If affects the three ascending dopaminergic systems and may explain many of the motor, emotional, affective and cognitive disorders associated with cerebral ageing. Senility and dementia affects the capacity for abstraction, conceptualization, reasoning, elaboration of strategies and problem solving, thus reflecting prefrontal deficiency symptoms. Aging along with depression, and lack of impulse control result from reduced nerve input (disafferentation) of the frontal lobe, when deprived of effective dopaminergic innervation.

The Uraeus is the head of the serpent, but the brainstem and spine is the tail of the cerebral Uroboros...by feeding the tail, we regenerate the head. Thus as we work to improve our sovereign cognitive powers through Uraeus and Heart-tree meditations and such...we also need to focus equally on increasing the energy, power, coherence, efficiency and bliss (*light*) of the brain stem itself. This will in turn have added benefits of improving digestion, cardiac and immune system function...and a general reduction in inflammation and aging. This is an ideal way to get rid of brain fog and restore higher cognitive capacity to the prefrontal lobes, due to the battery and roots of the brain being cleared and recharged. Focusing your meditations on the top of the forehead, encourages your disparate energies to coalesce to create a stream of creativity toward a goal. Syncing and linking the individual with the All, and allowing synchronicity to bring about serendipity and cocreative causatum.

• UNI-PHI/UNI-VERSE MEDITATION

I found this exercise during a live talk by *Nassim Haramein*. This meditation is for removing the veil of separation and reconnecting to the unified field through which all things are unified. All relationship becomes sacred when we Uni-phi with Uni-verse. In an infinitely energetic universe there is no shortage of energy, consciousness or love and so we never have to lack, we just have to learn how to harvest them. Making light or eating spin is a process of going within or interiorization into the stillness at the axle of rotation at the eye of the vortical torus of the **Merkabah**.

To Uni-Phi with Uni-Verse do the following steps:
- Stop the mind's self-reflexivity...the way it turns back onto itself.
- Decentralize awareness making the specificity and multiplicity one thing.
- Open the heart (8Hz) like a flower through breathing deeply into it..
- Relax the cells and reduce atomic "noise" –(zero inhibition of light)

- Warm one's field by radiating love – (remove darkness and fear)
- Give a total body smile at the atomic level – (Unification)
- Make love with the vacuum - (no separation)
- In this there can be no collapse of awareness recursively back into the past separate-self-sense – (radiant awareness)
- Then we see "reality" in pure awareness through the eyes of the universe observing itself. (cosmic consciousness)
- Healing involves moving the flow of energy, sensation and consciousness to promote greater feeding of matter with vacuum energy to increase spin.

The secret elixir of youth is doing the work that you love, following your passion. Inner sovereignty comes from the "Pure Heart" and yields perseverance, courage, resolve, endurance, composure and grace. Inner sovereignty amounts to the greatest gifts in life…character, nerve, substance and class. The deep inner strength and quiet determination of the Pure Heart reflects the power of geometry inherent in the Unified Field — there is no greater power in the Universe than the Unified Force. To see, know and be all things. That which is not tuned into Phi cannot be sustained, it is entropic, it is losing energy, money, consciousness, love, order etc…

The shift to a holy, whole, healthy culture requires the waking up from the nightmare of survival-of-the-most-evil, to the Reality of natural abundance and happiness for all. Vitality is not gained through egoic force and false stimulation that destroys the subtle Phi movement arising from the torque, the Coriolis effect, spin and the angular momentum of the spiraling nature of the spacetime manifold. By building the senses and neurology for communication with the Inner Man and the zeropoint source of Being we can become immune to the veil of terror propagated by the disenfranchised, power hungry Borg. You have to lose yourself to find yourself. Finding yourself means breaking with the unfulfilling patterns of the past, for the past conditioned self is not you anyway.

This competition thing, this conditioning which has been naively installed in the psyche of man is plainly suicide. We now know that cooperation has to be the pivot around which all human life centered or we would always be on the very edge of extinction—always living in fear of ourselves. Co-operation and co-creativity produce the kind of solidarity and fearlessness whereby the people can free themselves from extortion by the agents of psychopathic control. Unless each individual self-actualizes and discovers their true calling within the stream of genuine human progress then the whole is made less than. Through the Inner Arts we practice self-intimacy and thus achieve intimacy with all existence, to establish a sense of haunting and exhilarating wonder for the unfathomable mystery of the Universe.

It is an accretion of cultural figments, impressions and experiences largely imposed on a more passive and defensive sponge that is not yet self-deterministic. In order to gain self-dominion, Self-knowledge, gnosis and integrated Psi, mystic and visionary capacities, we must let the pupael self dissolve away. In the beginning stages of emerging from slave consciousness there is grief that occurs during the limbo period between acquiring the mastery of the sovereign self, and losing our higher self in the petty demands of daily life. Thus awakening is an act of surrender and faith, plus the building of the new, within the catabolic collapse of the old. Thus an individual's metamorphosis into the whole HUman is a metaphor for the process of cultural evolution as a whole, and it requires the pro-vision to see beyond The Given. To raise and maintain our charge and reconnect with cosmic resonance we must free ourselves from default programming and automatic, blind embeddedness in The Given cultural trance of centralized power.

• THE EMANCIPATOR

Activated and liberated energy (kundalini) opens, softens and integrates the body allowing for growth, evolution and awakening to a more profound experience of being HUman. The philosophy behind this invention is that the pelvis (first chakra) is the incoming faucet to God. That is, the base of the spine is the source and storage of the bodymind's energy prior to its movement up the spine and the higher levels of animal/human functioning. Therefore if the storehouse and origins of our energy is caged within a cemented, contracted and unconscious pelvis then there is less flow in the entire body-mind-soul complex.

This "ossification," depression and imprisoning of lifeforce means less energy is available for spiritual cultivation and creativity, and this translates as stagnation, repression and regression in the life of the individual, and fascist conservatism and depression in society at large. You can't integrate sexuality and sensuality by avoiding or damning it, and you can't evolve it by using and abusing it as a tool for Hindbrain power. Since sexuality/sensuality is the vital force it must be allowed to flow free in order to evolve and transmute life and flesh to the quintessence of the divine. Sexual suppression amounts to soul suppression, for there is but ONE energy, and that which is repressed cannot evolve.

The Emancipator is a tool that can be used to amplify sex in both the female on top, and female on bottom positions. The sex tool gives women that extra freedom and power to met her man with a more energetic thrust during sex and to not be passively pinned down. Not only will this liberate the pelvis and psycho-spiritual sexual energies of both partners, it will translate to more equality and intimacy between the sexes and in all aspects of relationship and society. As the woman becomes more of an active agent in bed she discovers her assertive, agentic powers for manifestation in the world at large. This sex tool uses physics and engineering principles to amplify sex, but its use is entirely intuitive and organic.

Email me at jananz@hotmail.com if you are an awake international online entrepreneur looking for the ultimate world changing product to generate billions for your cultural restoration projects.

Life cannot be pinned down, so there is no alternative but to set it free.

CHAPTER 5

FACILITATING THE INNER MARRIAGE

A Science of Bridges or an Evolutionary Science of the Remarriage of the Poles. This is a multidisciplinary integral science specifically for the purpose of investigating and making conscious the alchemy of subtle/causal level relationships and spiritual practice. Transpersonal Reality is the Land of Bridges or inclusion. Following are some Inner Arts for overcoming the various schisms caused by neglect, latency and trauma in order to substantiate the unified core-self. By integrating the bodymind and building sovereignty we learn to make self-nurturing decisions because we are in communication with our "Self." These practices are a continuation of the Inner Arts introduced in Biology of Kundalini. They slowly change the baseline brain state by using Neuroemotional kinesthetic-Sensory-Visual techniques to facilitate the inner marriage

• HEMISPHERIC INTEGRATION

Rapid shifting of the eyes side to side (EMDR—Eye Movement Desensitization Reprocessing Therapy), or any binaural therapy such as throwing an object from hand to hand, walking, or Emotional Freedom Technique (tapping) would help overcome the brain damaging effect of rejection and build confidence. Juggling, sticks, hula-hoops, and other dexterity challenges. Crossing over the body movement or body positions as well as art and dance would also help cover come the anesthetization of the central hemispheric cross communications and build up the efficiency of the corpus callosum. See the Inner Arts and Kundalini Skills on my website. Binaural music, especially the Sound of the Sun and water charged with the vibration of the Sound of the Sun.

• UPRIGHT WALKING

To change life patterns the body-brain we created in the past has to be restructured, or else the same behavioral and social patterns will still continue. Upright walking is one of the most effective ways of repatterning consciousness beyond defensive conditioning. Go for a walk and keep your eyes focused at eye height or higher, ie: you will be looking at treetops, roofs and sky. You may find this difficult at first but keep working into the position by easing out the kinks in your jaw, neck and shoulders. The upright position puts the head correctly on the spine, breathing is lower into the lungs, digestion is assisted and shoulders are naturally down and back. The brain is fed with more blood and oxygen and is able to detoxify and drain better, sinuses clear and the throat opens up to more energy and emotion. Dropping the back of the tongue and jaw opens the breath to oxygenate the brain more fully, doing the Inner Smile while upright walking helps maintain the alignment for ennobled-attraction

When first starting out with upright walking you will probably find you have to spend considerable energy and effort in the beginning to retrain your posture and metabolism. As resistance to change arises in the jaw, yawn those blockages away. It helps to emote or make sounds to break out of the Borg… ie: the more down trodden, head forward stance most of us normally walk around in. Pain may be felt in the facial muscles as they let go of their former set. Rub a thin film of Magnesium chloride liquid on your face, neck and shoulders prior to your walk; this will assist in the decontraction process.

"**Magnesium oil**" is Magnesium chloride that is Mg salt. Epsom salts also works as a spray, but is not as easily absorbed. If you put DMSO in it the Magnesium chloride penetrates deeper into the tissues. If you don't have DMSO you can use MSM to the same effect. Dimethyl sulfoxide (DMSO) is an organosulfur solvent which dissolves both polar and non-polar compounds. It is used for pain and inflammation and most often as a "transporter" for other constituents.

The longer your upright walking session the more lasting its influence will be on the rest of your life. If you do go for an epic upright walk, of say four or more hours, then have an Epsom salt bath directly afterwards to prevent muscle soreness. You will also notice the need to sleep more at the beginning of the upright practice as the restructuring becomes integrated at a deep level.

As we break out of our dog-beaten slave stance we stand up tall in the stream of life and recover higher, majestic levels of our humanity. The change in our brain chemistry magically creates a whole new life—as structure determines fate. For pineal health do not wear sunglasses on your walks but take some with you in case you have to walk towards the sun and have to be directly looking at it with your upright gaze. You will find it impossible to be depressed during an upright walk and if you do the Inner Candle at the same time, you can bathe in the perpetual honey of your own noble being in connection to nature. For this you must be outside and walking within the electromagnetic energy currents of earth and sky.

Since this posture increases energy to the brain you may feel unsettled and disorientated for a while afterward. If you continue with upright walking as a daily practice you will loose this sense of discomfort and establish a new equilibrium and personality reflecting a loss of hesitation, rigidity and increased Flow. As you move into Whole person functioning you will notice parts of you that were stagnant come alive and you will discover newfound gifts you didn't know you had.

Know that there is a light at the end of the tunnel and you will be bigger and more profound on reaching it, so trust in the process itself and do as you are informed by the energy of awakening itself. It means you have to embrace it, keep up your fortitude and stamina and keep an eye on the horizon (both objectively and subjectively). As your brain and head come alive, so too does your heart and the rest of your bodymind and soul as well. As the German philosopher Friedrich Nietzsche said that you should *"never trust a thought that didn't come by walking."* I say…never trust a thought that didn't come by upright walking!

• NEW THOUGHT WALK

Thinking gets repetitive when our energy is low. Those with under active thyroid, exhausted adrenals, fatigue and impaired metabolism may find they are constantly replaying old thought. To break the habit of regurgitating tired worn out mental patterns the blood needs to be moved, stimulated and oxygenated with exercise to remove the carbon dioxide and acid toxins, thereby improving cellular energy. Go for at least a half hour upright walk, using slightly exaggerated speed, gait and arm movements. When upright walking I find breathing through the mouth better to load the lungs with more air. As the stale thoughts come up, send them away immediately and repeat the mantra "New Thought." The New-Thought Walk is like a refresher course which disciplines your brain to find "old thought" distasteful and to remember it is devitalizing. When you think about it 99% of recycled thought is useless, and should be sent to the compost heap where it belongs. Thought regurgitation is a sign we are traveling downhill in a prolapsed, submerged, descended and unconscious state. This sunken condition is the opposite of the high energy, creative state that will actually take us wherever we actually want to go. If old stinking thinking arises just don't go there and focus on movement, oxygen and noble posture. Reality is "Ever New" and so should we be.

• NOBLE POSTURE

Upright walking is essential to the stabilization of sovereignty in everyday life in order to maintain our noble stature. This is so because the advanced human principle is tied into the wiring of our upright posture and the bipedal state. Also the liberation of our breathing in combination with the correct feeding of energy and oxygen to the brain reinforces the full incarnation of Presence. Plus the left/right leg movement enhances binaural communication between the hemispheres and aids whole brain integration. Awakening sovereignty is reliant on the perfect orientation of the head on the spine to allow the full flow of consciousness between brain and body, thus strength, flexibility and position of the spine and posture come into play as the foundations of the sovereign state. This is the simplicity of the core sovereignty teaching. The secret to charisma is regal bearing. Ideally, your body language should communicate Presence, strength, grace, competence, and command.

• BREATHING

We take 26,000 breaths a day, and if we start to have a conscious relationship with this aspect of existence we can live without stagnated emotional fears and energy depletion. If done correctly, each and every breath can be rejuvenating and invigorating. If you are not breathing fully and deeply from the belly then you are missing out on the fullness of your own being. Breathing and increasing the oxygen carrying capacity of the blood is the principle method of stress relief, stress prevention and allowing Higher Homeostasis. High oxygen levels are important to activate the neocortex, otherwise the reptilian and mammalian brain will be more dominant if there is a lack of oxygen in the body.

Deep breathing thus overcomes self-rejection, alienation, low self-esteem, negative emotions and disempowerment. There is no closer and more reliable resource for liberation available to us than breath, in enabling us to conquer ourselves and establish right relationship with the world. Breathing is key, but it is more a matter of oxygen flooding to penetrate thresholds, aerobic exercise and watching one's breathing pattern during the day and breathing deeper. Alternative nostril breathing is secondary to basic observation and expansion of one's daily breathing habits.

• CORE BREATHING

With hands on the belly…breathe in through the nose down into the belly. On the out-breath press onto the belly with the hands and clench abdominal muscles. In this way you tone the abs, improve digestion, oxygenate the brain and energize the bodymind. Core strength is important to sovereignty. Breathing in more oxygen elevates the synthesis of serotonin in the central nervous system, and alkalinizes and detoxifies the blood. The higher serotonin levels and correspondingly higher levels of motor activity in the dominant animals provides them with the means to take better advantage of their resource opportunities. Through breath we can overcome deflation, morbidity and retreat to respond positively to life-changes.

When you love and breathe without restraint, you maintain a balance of force that keeps your mind and body and spirit functioning and moving in a direction for growth and development. Through using breath to progressively wake up we can improve life satisfaction by engaging in joyous, unrestrained and enthusiastic planning of future activities. Breathing is the foundation of life and applied breath is essential to stabilize the mystic state and the life of the visionary. Shift your energy to a higher vibration by breathing slowly and deeply for 10 minutes to consciously change to a more empowered state.

• FISH BREATHING

Another type of regenerating breath that is good for stabilizing energy and integrating emotion during panic attacks or heart expansions is Fish Breathing. This is especially effective while walking upright, as I find breathing through the mouth better to load the lungs with more air. The mouth is completely relaxed and pursed like a fish. You circular breathe in and out of the mouth without pausing between the in and out breath. Make the in-breath nasally and the out-breath throaty. The continuous, non-pause breathing can be done through the nose also when needing more brain power during peak kundalini activity or peak concentration. This is not the musicians' circular breathing technique accomplished by breathing in through the nose while simultaneously pushing air out through the mouth using air stored in the cheeks. The word inspire is based on the roots "in" and "spire" or literally, to breathe in.

> . "Only that which is deeply felt can change us…rational arguments alone cannot penetrate the layers of fear and conditioning that comprise our crippling belief systems." Marilyn Ferguson.

• BELLOWS WALKING

While out walking, feel where in the body you are holding your fear…eg: in your diaphragm, or around the adrenals and the back of the heart. Then use your breath, breathing through the mouth, to pull the nectar of the heart into the area resonating in fear. Wisdom (ie: body-knowing) is found through purification of the frequencies of past patterns with the heart—to clean the mirror of the heart to embrace a "higher" reality. Use this technique in association with Upright Walking.

• WHO IS WALKING?

WHO is awake? WHO is real? In natural landscape in which you won't be heard do a deep throated toning of "WHO" with pursed lips in rhythm with your step. It feels a little gorilla-like. It cleans and balances the brain. Vibroacoustic stimulation of toning to vibrate the skull, cleaning cerebral spinal fluid, enabling better transmission of neural transmitters across the synaptic gaps and enhancing their re-uptake, as well as stimulating the pituitary's dissemination of hormones.

• SNIFF BREATHING WALK

Sniff breathing walk to clear the sinuses works to remove brainfog and focus the mind. Doing around 20-30 big sniffs while walking outside usually does it. Also steaming the face to stimulate lymph drainage from the head helps to remove congestion and stagnation. Also vigorously swishing the mouth with saline solution and saline nasal spray help to clear consciousness, as does tapping the jaw and neck with the mouth open. These are just a few tips that help lymphatic drainage from the head, however exercise is of primary importance.

• SEROTONIN, GROUNDING AND OXYGEN

The upright walking posture opens the rib cage and deeper breathing and greater massaging of the digestive system with each breath. The increased oxygen supply raises serotonin levels, which amplifies consciousness. Alpha animals have more serotonin in their system, and thus are calmer than subordinates. The ability to remain calm and confident under duress permits clearer thought in general and increases the expression of personal power, which raises our social status. More serotonin also improves digestion and protects against depression, allowing a more agentic and responsive approach to events. The calm of serotonin allows the neurological stability to facilitate greater brain differentiation and integration toward a more mature, empowered sovereign state. Oxygen levels in the brain are tied to levels of the neurotransmitter serotonin. You can regulate your levels of brain serotonin by controlling your breath. Too much serotonin in the brain causes irritation, tension, and stress. Dropping the levels of serotonin can result in greater relaxation and allow the brain's nonlinear activities to flow more smoothly and facilitate access to deeper intuitive, inspired layers of mind. To be inspired is to be full of the breath of life, Chi, Prana or Spirit. Mood elevating Ginkgo Biloba increases the brain uptake of serotonin.

• NEGATIVE ION AIR

When negative ions are inhaled and reach our bloodstream, they are believed to regulate levels of the mood chemical serotonin, consequently helping in alleviating depression, anxiety and stress, while also boosting our energy. Increasing the negative ion content of the air promotes alpha brain waves and increases brain wave amplitude. This produces ion induced alpha waves to spread from the occipital areas to the parietal and temporal, reaching the front lobes, spreading evenly across the right and left brain hemispheres. This creates an overall clear and calming effect, thus, promoting better concentration. Methods of increasing negative ions include purchasing an air ionizer for your home, open windows, water fountains, houseplants, Himalayan Salt lamps, H_2O kinetic™ shower heads, using natural building materials and natural fiber clothing.

• MAINTAINING PRESENCE

Presence is a term I use for the "felt-sense" of the full-sensory moment without resistance (push, pull, shove, retreat). You'll find it takes less energy to be in Presence than to be in the ego (Borg) because in the slumped condition we are parasitizing ourselves and therefore not in a reciprocal energy exchange nor synergistic relationship with our environment. When not we are not present our spine is bent, our diaphragm contracted, thus we are oxygen deprived with low brain energy and so thought habituates in well-trodden tracks. This hints to the fact that to wake up we need to straighten our spine, breathe more fully in order to become Present and live more fully. It takes significant energy and focus to become Present, but once there the energy circulation us and the EMF world is such that we can drop the low energy state of the Borg, for our subtle energy is being fed.

• TURNING THE HEAD TO THE LEFT

The suppression of the enteric brain (parasympathetic) is why we are presently a left brain dominant species. Reduced function and decreased metabolism in the left prefrontal cortex is linked to depression and worry. It is the left hippocampus that tends to store the preponderance of our narrative story, suggesting its invariant involvement in remembering autobiographical events throughout our lifespan. While the right hippocampus and dorsal amygdala may be responding specifically to recent autobiographical events that have a more positive emotive valence. Turning the head to the left switches off the emotional regurgitation of unpleasant current events that our defensive ego has gotten "stuck" on.

• CORE BUILDING

Lie on your back, left hand is over the right side of the heart in the center of the chest fingers pointing down to the right. Right hand is over your back between the scapula on the right side of the spine. Do the Inner Candle in this position; it is good to have a flickering candle going by the bed and be listening to music such as Jeffrey Thompson's Awakened Mind System.

• REPATTERNING

The self-protection trap gives us emotional constipation that makes it impossible to deal with our deeper feelings, and the result is that these feelings stay hidden and don't evolve or dissolve. Binaural music and meditation slows the brainwaves, increasing electrical fluctuations in the brain, changing the neural structure and allowing the brain to reorganize itself at a more complex higher level. Sungazing charges the brain core with photons and increases hemispheric synchronization, so it is advised during Neuroemotional Reprogramming repatterning periods as it one of the ultimate brain-wipe methods.

• CLICK AND DRAG

We perceive threatening events or feelings as "attacks" that we need to "defend" against. The easiest way to recall cut-off parts back into the whole is to energetically get the sense that you are moving the ego blockage, painful organ or emotional miasma over into the heart, and the heart will then spread its field out into the blocked, cut off area. *Gather that negative emotion, numbness or pain and click and drag it into your heart!* Where awareness goes energy goes—where energy goes blood goes—where blood goes life flows.

• COSMIC JELLYFISH

Lying on your stomach with the head to one side; do a mind-meld-two-pointer by pressing the thumb tip in the crook where the nose meets the eye brow and the index finger pointing up to press on the middle of the head just over the ridge of the forehead. Do the Inner Candle while in this position and drop your whole body relaxing it completely into a jellyfish state. Turn your head and do the same thing on the other side.

• ORMUS, MOOD, WATER AND LIGHT

The Alpha Learning Institute of Switzerland found that these m-state, monatomic elements improve nerve coherency and hemispheric synchronization, thereby raising intelligence, creativity, bodymind coordination, agility, eliminating depression and reducing stress! Taking *Orbitally Rearranged Monatomic Elements* (ORMUS) during awakening is a way to speed metadaptation, reduce nerve damage, provide free radical protection and detoxification, regulate brain activity and strengthening brain wave coherence.

www.subtleenergies.com —Barry Carter's ORMUS site.

• TURNING OFF AND TUNING IN

By dropping the muscles at the back of the tongue, this puts you into throaty belly breath, and along with the endorphin generating Inner Smile this will immediately turn on the parasympathetic nervous system. Always look for the fulcrum point in physiology to effect change, by treating your body as though it is a mechanical temple you are exploring. The fulcrum point for removing tension from the jaw is to relax the muscles at the back of the tongue and put on the Inner Smile. As you do this imagine the tongue dropping into the belly for infinity. The jaw simply won't relax without doing this, for you have to access the Vagus Nerve and turn on the nervous system's parasympathetic off switch. The PTSD body has been wired by trauma, so often considerable effort is needed to tone the sympathetic side down enough to balance the two sides of the central nervous system. This reharmonizing is the main job at the beginning spiritual practice to fully embody the physical house of the soul.

Presence requires high energy, photons, conductivity, oxygen and free electrons, thus an exercised-remineralized raw body, lying on the earth in the sun while deep breathing is the combination by which we can unlock the vault of incarnation and begin to "show up" no matter what past hells we have endured that make us want to retreat into oblivion. To start off the deep opening of the jaw you can use a little harmine oil on the jaw itself. Syrian rue/cinnamon/galangal heating oil can also be used for relaxing the jaw via harmine. GABA, the body's main inhibitory (calming) neurotransmitter, stimulates the production of Human Growth Hormone (HGH). Valerian, jatamansi, L-Pyroglutamic Acid, SAMe, vitamin B6 and green tea increase GABA.

• THE QUANTUM BATH

Difficult symptoms and ill health is simply inferior subatomic, molecular, cellular, neurological, EMF and light connection. Improve the bodymind structure, function and communication flow and what you now experience as demons, become the Daemon, the Muse, the Holy Spirit or Presence. According to Jung, if we follow the inner voice of our Muse we will find our true vocation, snap out of our neurosis and heal our suffering.

If we sustain the frequency of health long enough we become healthy. There is a saying that we must "believe" in love! Well to be healthy we must "believe" in health by feeling what that is on the cellular level apriori to disease. Through conditioned responses to the world, in presovereign humans the head brain suppresses the enormous pain of self-neglect and self-abuse in the solar plexus brain. Dropping the repressive mode requires higher frequency entrainment via the quantum mind or space brain, where there is no "cognitive content." It involves getting rid of the sadness in the lungs, and closure of the throat and putting the minds eye in the solar plexus, while breathing into the belly. Then focusing peace into the brainstem when the pain in the solar plexus presents itself.

• THE PISS BATH

Druing Kundalini Awakenings or extreme stress the piss bath is guaranteed to lower high blood pressure and helps clear glutamine excitotoxicity in the brain by triggering the kidneys to produce the urinating hormones and the blood vessel relaxer vasopressin. Make a hot bath with 2 cups of Epsom Salt and essential oils or herbs. Put on atmospheric music (such as alpha or theta wave by Jeffrey Thompson, light candles and soak. Put hands on solar plexus, drop muscles at the back of the tongue and establish the Inner Smile. Breathe throatily down into the belly. Toning Huuuuu is also useful for brain cleansing, integration, relaxation and oxygenating. Urinate 3 times before leaving the bath; this takes at least an hour. This shows blood pressure is now lowered by changes of hormones in the kidneys. The knot in the solar plexus (the void of non-being) is dissolved by focusing peace and presence into the brainstem. This establishes higher connection between the head and the stomach brains whereby we have greater access to emotional intelligence, intuition and peace-celebration.

• EMOTIONAL SELF REGULATION

You can get rid of chronic emotional pain immediately if you reach into your inner parents, (the beneficent entity residing in your prefrontal lobes) and direct its calming, compassionate attention into the 2 year old having a tantrum in your belly. Only you can flip the switch and stop the unnecessary suffering with focused breathing. If you continue to abuse yourself with inner pain you will just find more reasons to suffer, for the world will move away from you, as people instinctively know they can do nothing for you if you yourself cannot regulate your own emotional state. Freedom and maturity is the self-determinacy to choose our own emotional state. The presovereign lets circumstances and social conditions determine their emotions, thoughts and behaviors. While a sovereign cultivates thought and emotion to uplift conditions, circumstances and social environment.

• EXECUTIVE PARENTING

Self leadership is transpersonally inspired from the Heart-prefrontal lobe connection to feed the human continuum. The soul is more realized and the personality more actualized when sovereign self-leadership is achieved. With sovereign parenting the true archetype of the soul is unveiled. Besides stewardship values of love, holding, nurturing, structuring, focusing, celebrating, allowing, and," we need discipline or strength of consciousness derived from gnostic integration to bring light into any darkness.

Stewart Swerdlow, a linguist who speaks ten languages, says that the often considered "unused" 90% portion of the brain is actually in constant communication with the Mind of God, receiving information in the Language of Hyperspace, a universal and interspecies language which consists of color, tone, and archetype. It is the transpersonal aspect of the sovereign that both directs and sustains the individual to support the continuum, for when we live eternity in the moment we effortlessly choose that which most awakens and furthers Life's cause. Gaining such automatic self-assurance, and self-reliance allows us the innate responsibility that is the source of the sovereign's capacity for freedom.

• RIDING SOLAR STORMS

Increased solar activity equates with an increased activation of your own personal Chi field, so you can use solar max and flares for your own ascension. Solar storms are useful to ride for repatterning one's life and removing what is not working, while making quantum jumps towards what you do want. Feed yourself with the increased energy of the solar storm rather than dissipating it in busy activity by doing Inner Arts like the Meditation for Attraction.

Simple adaptations for X-Class solar flares coming our way: Grounding-lie on the earth if possible, drink more water, reduce acid pH in body with fresh vege juice, avoid extra coffee, oxygen-conscious breathing, take negative ion walks in forest, river, ocean, take more B complex/Vitamin C/antioxidants/krill oil-Omega 3, Lecithin in smoothie. Go lite; avoid eating heavy cooked food-especially trans and heat damaged fats, increase raw-green in diet. Take kelp, Lygol's iodine drop in water; miso soup, spicy Thai food. Stretch and take hour long Epsom salt baths. Clay on the inside will also help integrate EMFs. Mud baths, clay packs and soaking in mineral water springs. I want to build stone igloos with mud baths for people to soak in to alternate darkness soaking with sun-gazing and sun-baking, back and forth for days or hours. For those you are undergoing a kundalini awakening, are highly stressed or unstable taking some radiation herbs during solar storms and solar max will help lessen the incoherence and dishevelment.

The sovereign is nothing if not causal with regards to their lens of perception and their responses. Our "job" as sovereigns is to make regeneration ubiquitous for there is far greater abundance to be made in life than in death. Growth has a subterranean building period where effects are not yet readily apparent then things become consciously apprehended, assimilated and transcended.

The higher your spin rate (the more energy the body has) the greater the sense of reality beyond the Flatland linear time of the material realm of the Borg. That is, the more enlightened (light flow or consciousness) we are the deeper our sense of perception into Timelessness or Eternity, Spiral time of the movement of the planetary Spheres of the solar system, **Kairos** or God's time-the mythic sense of time and timing associated with the archetypal symbolic mind and the collective unconscious. Thus during a kundalini awakening the psychic penetration of time through visions, dreams, precognition, synchronicity, telepathy, bio-navigation, lunar magnetism, solar gnosis can be overwhelming at times, unless one is able to assimilate this expanded time sense as "normal," or rather the supernatural and supratemporal as being the new normal.

The challenge of the Grand Solar Minimum and the magnetic reversal will test and expand our "sanity and survival" to breaking point. The energy from the Heliosphere Magnetotail explosions travel back along the field lines and BLAST the polar vortex down towards the equator, creating dangerously cold conditions, at the same time as a potential power outage. We must be aware that an EMP event caused by the sun can occur at night from these Matter:Antimatter spacegasms, and we can anticipate them by watching the coronal holes on spaceweather.com in combination with the heliosphere patterns on SWMF-RCM. The animated maps to follow are the SWMF 2011+ RCM Magnetosphere - BATSRUS - Y-CUT Magnetic Field Lines.
See: https://iswa.gsfc.nasa.gov/IswaSystemWebApp/

Check out my paper on these heliotail matter/antimatter explosions, as it is these rather than CMEs which will be affecting us during the current Grand Solar Minimum.
www.academia.edu/38222458/HELIOTAIL_PLASMA_EXPLOSIONS.pdf

CHAPTER 6

NECK AND THROAT

• THE PRIMAL SCREAM

The scream impulse goes right into the Dura matter or the thin membrane that is the outermost layer of the meninges that surround the brain and spinal cord. I felt this once during a Rosen Method session when a very painful kriya contraction went slowly up from the solar plexus through the core of my chest and neck and right into my skull. I interpreted it as a silent primal scream of un-released stored charge of trauma. I wonder what would happen if we brought back scream therapy. Through expressing what was repressed Arthur Janov argues that neurosis caused by the repressed pain of childhood trauma can be relieved by Primal therapy, through accessing the source of Pain within the more autonomic parts of the central nervous system. *The Primal Scream. Primal Therapy: The Cure for Neurosis* is a 1970 book by Arthur Janov.

• LIBERATING YOUR AUTHENTIC VOICE

Noble speech springs forth from the Heart. We must loosen up to break through into the sovereign state to speak with our authentic voice—for the rigid nescient self is prepersonal and presovereign, it is associated with the conditioned imprints we laid down through our interactions with everyone we ever met, and especially those in the first 0-3 years of our life. To find and re-connect with your authentic voice requires toning, breathing and aerobic exercise to establish Flow. Rolfing, or sexual healing workshops with your own gender gets the throat burning and pulsating open. Try the chopping wood exercise also (see kundalini skills list). You might try actively engaging novelty, change and travel to realize the the insubstantiality of your reality constructs, to get in touch with Kairos or divine synchronicity.

Detoxifying the old is necessary for establishing authentic, exuberant self-expression, which means stopping the numbing habits and energy leaks. It might also require some threshold penetrating shamanic allies like Ayahuasca, Iboga, trance dancing, Vipassana, fasting in nature, ORMUS initiation or adventures. We can establish an annual cycle associated with the moons and seasons of detoxification, perturbation, altered states, skill building, novel experience, personal challenge, service, vision-questing. In this way we treat each year like a hero's journey, so that over the course of our life our epic hero's journey becomes ever more conscious, precise and perfected. When starting to liberate your authentic voice put a note on your mirror with *"Take Your Cue"* written on it, and repeat the words mantra-style while walking.

• HYPER-EXTENDING THE THROAT

If you get a large broomstick and put your hands over one end of it with the other end poking into the ground by your feet, you can use the stick as a fulcrum for hyper extending your arms. With one foot in front of the other, you can hyper-extend your neck to stretch the throat and elongate the back in a swan-like pose. The head thrown back simultaneous with the pulling of shoulder/arms acts to emotionally open up the thyroid-throat area, thereby releasing sadness and silencing. For a singer, if you scrunch your legs down further into the Primal Release Pose around your ears, and try and breathe, moan and grunt or whatever down in that pose, this will unblock the diaphragm still further, but always remember to lie flat on your back afterwards to reset the brain toward relaxation of the body-cage.

• OPENING THE THROAT

We can open the throat by making peace (sympathetic resonance) in the brainstem. The eyeballs are turned back and down to the brainstem and silently say "peace" along with the breath; this allows intimate connection with the solar plexus brain, or soul-center - the source of life, light, and power, to the human body. Once the solar plexus brain is calmed and "included" then the throat is made available to conscious felt-sense, or inward bodily attention. When we first move into the throat area it may be in great dissonant distress if we have been holding onto our trauma from childhood. The child is not allowed or unable to voice their truth or their suffering and so it gets permanently caught and stored in the body. With hands on the throat and the heart, tone with the breath and continue focusing peace into the brainstem. This helps liberate the painful angst in the throat. In meeting the reality of the body's unhappiness we must not back away from it, but go into it.

The throat is one of the last places to open due to repressed metabolism (thyroid) and breathing, in combination with the systemic self-betrayal we must endure in our families of origin, schools, and authoritarian social institutes. Taking iodine and thyroid support nutrients, DHEA hormone and increasing the cells voltage and oxygen utilization helps to free the throat area. But it takes releasing sadness from the lungs and allowing joy to rise in the core, coupled with the sense of letting oneself go, regardless of social convention. This takes trance dancing, singing, outrageous vocalization and a safe place to be oneself, a space for letting the repressive mechanisms go.

The more we do this the more we can carry freedom into our daily lives, which in turn liberates those around us from their own repressive madness and conformity to mediocrity. The have to stabilize a certain level of apriori pleasure in being in order for the thyroid to relax and the throat to open. The Inner Arts with the mind's eye focus on the throat and allowing joy to bubble up from the belly and the lungs can be applied to facilitate the ongoing opening of our main blockage to truth communication.

• RELEASING THE JAW

It takes years to get kundalini through the jaw because of the left-brain betawave overdrive of the culture that forces us into a chronic stress response to our daily lives. The tiger never really does go away, and we never fully relax even while we sleep. In a presovereign culture we carry on jaw tightness from childhood, which is basically fossilized silence from not being able to speak our truth and speak out about injustice, abuse and shaming. Then the pyramid power system in work and financial class keeps the jaw rigidity intact throughout adult life.

As long as the jaw holds onto its fossil tension the prefrontal lobes cannot fully commune with the heartfield, thus preventing wholebrain consciousness. Releasing the fossil tension will bring temporary relief, but the only way to find permanent relief is to retrain the posture of the whole body. The skull must be supported by correct pelvic alignment to take the stress off of the head, neck and shoulders, thus allowing the skull to float at the top of the spine and the jaw to release. Upright walking encourages the correct stature for a supported skull and relaxed jaw—to train yourself simply balance a book on top of your head.

The jaw is released by building peace in the brainstem, alkalinizing and oxygenating the blood, melting it with sun heated iron-rich rocks, and grounding of the jaw on the grass or sand. Learning to use your true voice, rebirthing breathing, float tanks, gestalt and social expression, sexual healing workshops, bodywork and the arts will help rewire the brain to have more balance between the sympathetic and parasympathetic sides of the autonomic nervous system and reduce the inertia waste of energy caught in the jaw and other armor blockages. In the bath do the Heart-tree Meditation connecting the solar plexus to the throat while toning Toning Huuuuu is also useful for brain cleansing, integration, relaxation and oxygenating. The wholebrain stance that permits the sovereign state is to drop the muscles at the back of the tongue and establish the Inner Smile, while breathing throatily into the belly. Ultimately doing these three things throughout the day will permanently rewire the brain to be more dual hemisphere, while drawing on the heart and the solar plexus brains.

Basically without fully integrating both hemispheres, the heart and the solar plexus brains, we are NOT in growth and thrival mode (love), we are in force and survival mode (fear). Speaking one's truth is difficult if one has to work for a living, because those with greater authority inevitably use shaming slights and digs to "get at one" for the simple reason that subordinates cannot speak out against injustice. This kind of abuse is a form of sexual harassment because it is the same dopamine, adrenalin mix that the attacker is after when they inflict moral injustice, or paranoic defamation, and malicious talk on those further down the pyramid. Power-abuse is the number one addiction of the human species, and it will be its ultimate downfall because it is degenerative and anti-evolution. .

Every instance of negative power contributes to the ongoing downfall of humanity.

• GET LOUD!

To rectify our dopamine receptors and epigenetics from the anti-developmental effects of trauma and neglect it is necessary to work against the closure processes of self-diminishment, self-negation, numbing and nullification. Thus it helps to engage in LOUD therapy and activity that expands the sense of self to gargantuan proportions. We can push back against self-closure by exaggerated loud speech, singing, animal noises and screaming combined with vigorous, aggressive body movements and exercises that expand the range of the body. Novel self-expression, body sensation, experiences and new movements also help to reinstate the basic integrative wiring between the motor cortex, limbic system and the executive brain, overcoming the standing pattern of the hijacking of the brain by the amygdala that paralyses and stagnates the flow of being by locking the brain into the "defensive" mode rather than the "growth" mode.

We are ALL refugees transitioning from the death culture to the vital-living culture. Besides regular sports, other methods for increasing a powerful expression of self-will includes *"pushing against"* such as wrestling, rolling on tennis balls, arm exercises, rowing, and isometric pressing against walls, door frames etc...with all body parts. It is now understood that fascial network is one of our richest sensory organs. The proprioceptive cells affecting our muscles, are not in the muscle, but in the **fascia** surrounding the muscle bundles. Stretching and isometric pressing exercise makes the body more conscious by strengthening the fascial light body through which superluminal information flows. The ultimate exercise for the diaphragm and Gate of Life release exercise is The Primal Release Pose, which gets to the neurological heart of somatic shame, grief and social stress.

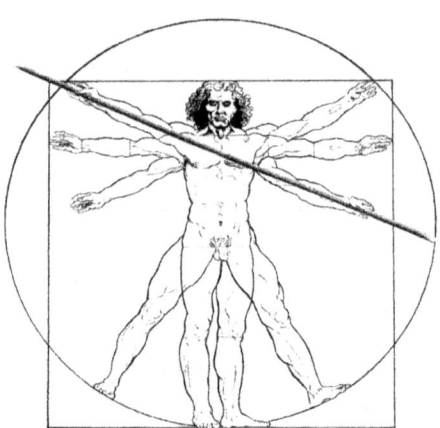

A curtain rod can be used for Vitruvian Man 360° stretches of the maximum self-boundary, so that the fascia is stretched and made subtle and open to the flow of light. By expanding the boundaries of the self we give ourselves room and licence to be as big as we can be.

CHAPTER 7

HEALING THE SPINE

"The whole body is rooted in the spine. If the spine is young, you are young. If the spine is old, you are old. If you can keep your spine young, it is difficult to become old. Everything depends on your spine. If your spine is alive, you will have a very brilliant mind. If the spine is dull and dead, you will have a very dull mind. The whole of yoga tries in many ways to make your spine alive, brilliant, filled with light, young and fresh." Osho, Meditation: The First and Last Freedom

Keeping the spine open and flexible is essential to full utilization of the brain's capacities. Loosening the spine and joints to improve flexibility really helps to get the neuro-juices flowing. Body armor is the physical correlation to neurosis and psychosis and all pathology, which is a symptomatic of dehumanization. By spinal yoga I refer to various methods of opening, enlivening and regenerating the spine, such as Primal Release Pose, ball rolling, hanging, flexing, spinal rebirthing, spinal shower and earthing on the grass. The top and bottom of the spine must be opened at the same time for they are opposite ends of one unified system of energy flow.

• SPINAL OPENING

You are as young as your spine is open! To remove scoliosis and calcification in the spine you need to up your magnesium intake and use Epsom salts in the bath. Wheatgrass juice and raw greens are vital. Mineral supplementation with kelp, blue-green algae and leafy greens and weeds. Mega dose Vitamin C and Papaya/Pineapple enzymes while you are restructuring. Sunbathe nude to allow the sun to catalyze deposit removal and correct restructuring. Drink 4 qts of water per day. Hang by the hips for 3 minutes several times per day. Walk barefoot in nature and lie on the ground. Bury yourself in sand for a few hours. Use a plastic roller ball for spinal rolling several times per day along with the Primal Release Pose. The spinal shower is the ultimate spinal healing devise. Watch "David Wolfe on Calcium" on youtube.

• SPINAL REBIRTHING

I had a dream that I did a spinal extension technique on a young woman who had been affection deprived in childhood. She crouched on the ground (in a squat position on her feet with hands on the ground in front) and I put my hands on either side of her spine at the back of her chest. She pressed up into my hands, while I pressed down against her. Her spine cracked about 10 times. Starting off at the lower back and then moving the hands up to finally press up by the shoulders.

This spinal compression/extension can be used at the bottom of the spine by pushing up into a therapists hands with the legs. In the middle of the spine by pushing up on all fours and at the top of the spine by pushing up with the arms. It is the most cathartic and radical form of spinal release I have found. Its effectiveness may be based on the fact that contraction can be released by overextending already contracted muscles, so that when the brain sends its relaxation signal the muscles let go further than they were originally. Emotionally the burden is lifted once the tension is acknowledged, rather than carrying the load around for years, making the body numb with pain and very inefficient, debilitated and ineffectual. With spinal rebirthing we "feel" into the numbness and recover what was lost to us due to the freeze response.

• THE SPINAL SHOWER

Water therapy, or moving mineral water and sunlight is best way to heal from PTSD and childhood trauma. Hence the spinal shower! You can remove multigenerational trauma from the nervous system with the spinal shower. The Spinal Shower is the one true method of achieving profound cellular gratitude by giving the bodymind maximum release from accumulated toxicity (depolarization).

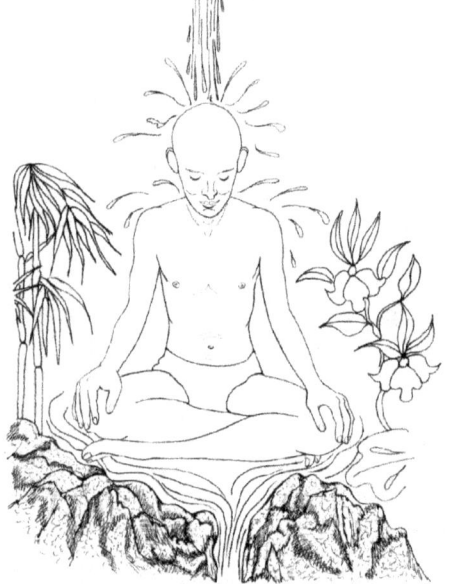

The ultimate healing devise is a 3" column of water falling about 4 feet onto the head and spine is I think the most profound releaser, detoxifier and opener of the central nervous system. Allowing "growth," that is a deeper synthesis of consciousness and higher neurological integration to occur. The pain that is released is the latency and abuse of a conscious creature living in an unconscious culture. As the tension in the neuromuscular system is felt it is released, thereby permitting greater incarnation and integration. It was the most painful experience I have had because it touches the very heart of our "holding," the pain is exquisite. With a continuous stream of warm water we can move through *"the pain of separation"* and touch the self-neglect and self-abandonment in our tissues…to become spiritually organic and alive again. It has radical effects in "unconditional meeting" and eliminating stored pain and emotion. While sitting under this flow one goes into a deep trance, facilitating healing of both the muscular and nervous system at the deepest level. I also think a sensory-maximization-super-spa with hundreds of jets may work to release fossilized tension. The great thing about water flow is that it is chaotic; this arrhythmic flow helps to break up structure and resistance.

• HANGING

Hanging from the hips over a bar 10 minutes a day is the best place to "start" our kundalini skills practice. I think it the most significant factor in "sustaining" a de-contraction progress. The benefits of hanging include: general pick-me-up, higher consciousness mode, forward momentum, opens the pelvis to grounding energy from the earth, elongates spine, feeds the brain, harmonizes sympathetic/parasympathetic sides of nervous system, stimulates blood/lymph/O_2, increases metabolism. The bar should be about 2" diameter; put a towel over it for padding; hang from the hips with both the arms and legs hanging free off the ground. Start off at 5 minutes in the morning, and 5 in the late afternoon or so. Do not do handing during major heart expansion periods, or during times of high blood pressure in the head associated with sympathetic nervous system hyperactivation.

• SWAN POSE

Stand like the Maiden on the Prow of a ship, arms held back by clasping the hands behind you, chest radically protruding and breathe deeply into this pose. Breathe in through the crown chakra and out through the solar plexus. Adopting this stance as a general living posture will change ones wiring and life in short order. It especially helps overcome the sexual harassment, the shaming and victimhood of living in this culture as a woman, and for powerlessness in general

• SOLAR SPHINX POSE

The Solar Sphinx pose uses "unconditional" light radiating out from the core sun to cleanse the push-pull of self/other in order to be a pure vessel for relationship beyond the automatic patterns of attraction and aversion arising from imprints. Sit with your back against a wall or tree, knees pulled up close to the chest. Put hands between thighs and touch fingertips together in a solid wakeful press. Imagine you are sitting in a Merkaba (Chariot of Ascension) that is a 3D star tetrahedron of a married upright and down triangle. Feel the center of the Merkaba at the core of the body between the spine at the 12th thoracic and the solar plexus. Imagine rays of light pouring forth from this internal sun. Now turn the minds eye up to generate the Uraeus and sustain the serpent's head as an emergent extension out of the top of the forehead.

Drop tongue and deepen breathing as usual for sovereignty exercises. Shift awareness between Merkaba, internal sun, finger press and Uraeus until you can comfortably keep all in your mind's eye at once. This practice builds integration and lessens anxious tension in body's core, generating coherence of light. The Merkaba is the vehicle for experiencing the eternal in the temporal world and allows the union of body, mind and soul. Such unification is what the symbol of the sphinx means.

• THE SPINAL YOGA ROLLER

This is an exercise ball used to provide support and resistance to compression for spinal rolling and as a fulcrum for leg-ups, scissors, diagonal pelvic twists, adrenal massage and other floor exercises. The sausage roll shape is far superior to the round exercise "ball" shape for stability, body cradling and for shifting positions around the body (exercise play/dance). Purchase from www.tantrapillow.com

Wilhelm Reich believed that cultural happiness in general and sexual happiness in particular are the real content of human life. The emotional abuse that contributes towards the armored bodymind is ultimately analogous to sexual abuse!, for the psychoneurosis generated by power-threat and shaming reduces sexual fulfillment and relational potential, and the capacity to enjoy life. In this way the fascist power-pyramid maintains itself through reducing sovereignty, original thought, creativity, joy and fulfillment of the real content and meaning of human life. We just have to love enough to not abandon the Self…then we can real-eyes spirit on earth. When we have a Wilhelm Reichian style re-evolution of the human species, only then are coexistence, inclusivity and celebration of diversity possible.

The work of regeneration aims to start first with the body and the earth to prepare the vessel for genuine spiritual growth, so we can move beyond mere socially adopted knowledge to ignite the cosmic genius within. Regeneration begins with opening and destagnating the body first, tuning the mind, body and relationships back toward biophilia or a love of Life and Lifeforce. The methods of transformation have to involve actual practice, they have to be enjoyable, and they must be appropriate to the needs and readiness of the times. To know the Self is to become integrated beyond mere learned knowledge. A "whole" person is the integration of mind, body and soul. This is the journey of transcendence of the external world and the beginnings of the truly spiritual life.

Meditation in a bodymind that is not in sync is merely a palliative that feeds the ego, but not the life of the Spirit. The more coherent the flow of communication within the higher the perspective achieved. The Transpersonal or Sovereign Worldview affords periscopic vision of the lens of perception permitting a wide field of view, allowing observation from a position displaced from a direct line of sight, giving distinct vision obliquely, or on all sides.

CHAPTER 8

HEALING THE HEART

Bliss is the plasma of the Heart's desire imploded into the vortical spin of the light in the body's informational forms.

The heart is the capacitor and field generator for the Merkaba or light vehicle of the body. **The Merkaba**, or etheric field, represents the full power of health and spiritual attainment of the individual. Love is the magnetic reconnection of polar opposites in sympathetic resonance. The magnetic reconnection of two colliding flows of plasma produces rapid and global changes to the arrangement of magnetic field lines; an efficient mechanism to convert energy stored in the magnetic field to kinetic energy producing an outflow of highly energetic particles, or "Love." At the center of the heart is an X-shaped transition region, with a 'separatrix' region that divides the in-flowing plasma vortices from the out-flowing vortices of highly energetic electromagnetic waves, which produces scalar waves, able to propagate over long distances, as in Global telepathy.

The greater the quantum coherence of the heartfield, the greater the love and the more perfect the instantaneous telepathic communication. The power of the heart goes up and down according to the vegetative annual solar cycle, the moon phases, the sunspot cycle, the weather etc... It also precognizes and arranges meetings with significant others, and draws people together via biomagnetism and nonlocal effects. The heart is superluminal and transtemporal, and mutliplexival in its consciousness, its senses and its emotion.

Any energetic, biochemical, physical or psycho-emotional blockage in the body diminishes the integrity of the heartfield. If the heartfield is compromised this reduces our capacity to love, and diminishes wholebrain consciousness and our capacity for cosmic connection (spirituality). In this disconnected state we are always maladapted and a victim to circumstances and our environment. Thus we see that sovereign empowerment is the ABSENCE of blockage to communication of consciousness and energy.

Consciousness, energy and matter are essentially ONE THING. Therefore there is no way of denying the fact that sacred society is only achieved through the sovereignty of each individual, and a culture that prevents this, is cosmically corrupt or evil (working against Eros). Besides the deep-rooted, ossified obstruction of the Borg pelvis which impedes the primordial energy at the base of the body's EMF egg, it is the jaw tension that manacles the upper end of the EMF egg and interrupts the vital charge and the amplitude, magnitude, expanse, holding power, quality, range and reach of our Merkaba.

The energy/consciousness conductivity of the sex/pelvis is a reflection of the condition of the throat jaw complex and vice versa. This is why sexual abuse in childhood invariably causes mouth, jaw, and tooth problems associated with the "silencing" of the individual's capacity to speak their truth. When truth is silenced so too is sacred sexuality, for sacred sexuality and truth go together or not at all. In a sense we should be calling lovemaking, "truth-making," for love is Truth! The full marriage, meeting or conjugation of charge. Patriarchal religions have misused the sexual and spiritual energy of the people for their own perverted games of war, plunger and tyranny. Anything that interferes with Eros, truth and the Christos is a form of torture in one form or another even if we are not conscious of the fact yet, and may never be.

You can't integrate sexuality/sensuality by avoiding or damning it, and you can't integrate it by using and abusing it as a tool for Hindbrain power. Since sexuality/sensuality is the vital force it must be allowed to flow free in order to evolve and transmute life and flesh to the quintessence of the divine. Whether or not you use sexuality/sensuality in relationship with other humans is irrelevant to the fundamental spiritual necessity of opening up the energetic faucet to God. In this brutal military-capitalist civilization, men's bodies have been abused, shamed, used, exploited and traumatized just as much as women — or there would not be so much insanity, war and dysfunction in the world. Pumping up boys on steroids and drugs to go shoot people in other countries for their resources is just one obvious betrayal of the masculine.

Thus those who ARE LOVE can love. This is the beauty of going raw, because only RAW is Real, and if we don't base our atomic existence in Universal Eros, then we are dying even as we strive ceaselessly to survive. Thrival requires exposing the lie of Thanatos and following the call of Eros towards an ever more illustrious understanding of life in the universe.

Emancipation Unlimited has many dearmoring products for removing the cage of contraction. The love-removal machine created by the brutal hysterical history of humanity is embedded in our neurological and genetic makeup, normalizing trauma and impinging on our capacity as superconscious beings. We all have ancestral trauma from humanity's violent past in our flesh and our DNA, and it is our responsibility as sovereigns and global citizens to free the spirit from its contracted cage. The hierarchal social structure and pyramid systems (predatory capitalism and resource wars) are keeping our collective enlightenment in the dumps. We must ceaselessly strive to take the lid off of our creative energy by restructuring our physiology, to find our way out of the cultural cul de sac. This is not an idle wish, it is a survival imperative, for in our current collective retardation and ignorance we are plainly suiciding the planet. Ignorance is darkness! So let there be light!

Peace is unity-love-flow or connectivity to All. Peace is arrived at by breaking out of the shell of defensive social conditioning. When the Borg is "undone" then peace reigns.

• HOLOGRAPHIC HEART-FIELD

The heart is a capacitor of the nondestructive compression of charge, condensing and attracting charge and receiving voltage from gravity. This constructive interference generates energy, bliss, heat, healing and consciousness. The implosion torsion field effect of heart expansion is the physics of enlightenment, involving nested fractal harmonics of the self-re-entry of recursive charge. We can use the heart-field as a vacuum cleaner to dissolve all miasmic and discordant frequencies (distortion, separation, disconnection) into the Zeropoint field. We become disgruntled (ungrounded) if we have not integrated the duality and multiplicity through the merger with the underlying ground of all being. In the stillness of the Void our fracturing and conflict are redeemed and unified in the underlying ground. By expanding the heart-field we can release all contraction, pain, blockage, numbness, emotional strain or tension and helplessness. Lie down on your back and breathe in through the top of the heat and send the out-breath down to form coriolis spirals in the pelvis. Use this energy to expand the möbius of the heart field and pour any suffering or holding into the field, such that the bodymind extends to infinity and you loose your sense of solidity. Infinite freedom is Love without measure.

• WHOLE BRAIN CONSCIOUSNESS

Whole brain consciousness is particularly reliant on flavonoids, especially in gaining access to the right brain, overcoming left-brain dominance and reducing inflammation (noise) in the brain. Over 4000 structurally unique flavonoids have been identified in plant sources. Acerola cherries, currants, camu-camu, tropical guava, grapefruit, kiwifruit, lychee, mulberries, oranges, cantaloupe, papaya, persimmons, elderberries and goji berries are all naturally rich in the full vitamin C complex and flavonoids. Saffron and other high flavonoid fruits and vegetables help to remove aluminum from the brain and reduce inflammation.

Flavonoids also have a major part to play in the hormones, neurotransmitters and gene expression. Moreover, flavonoids have protective actions in relation to abiotic stresses and also have anti-carcinogenic properties. Of the many actions of flavonoids, antioxidant and anti-proliferative effects stand out. Moreover, the inhibitory action on inflammatory cells, especially mast cells, appears to surpass any other clinically available compound.

The heart is the principle organ of wholebrain consciousness. The heart needs to be fed with Taurine, Omega-3, magnesium, cinnamon, kelp, greens, weeds, sprouts, berries and colorful fruits and veges. Romaine lettuce, asparagus, artichoke, arugula, kale, Swiss chard, collard greens, turnip/beet greens, sesame leaves, basil, parsley, mint, broccoli, cabbage, garlic mustard, brussels sprouts, green onions, leeks, spinach, zucchini, lambsquarters, thistle, and dandelion are the very best foods for your heart and blood vessels.

Lie on the grass a lot and go barefoot for earthing, the heart is both and electromagnetic organ, and a quantum implosion devise, so it needs a lot of nature in order to be whole. If you drop the muscles at the back of the tongue, put on an inner smile and do throaty breathing this links up the heart and solar plexus with the brain, balances the hemispheres, and takes you out of left-brain/Betawave overdrive.

• HEARTMATH ATTITUDINAL BREATHING

Focus on the heart on the in-breath and on the solar plexus on the out-breath. Choose a positive emotion such as gratitude, devotion, happiness joy, peace, forgiveness, care, courage or ease. Breathe the attitude in through the heart and out into the solar plexus. http://www.heartmath.org/research/our-heart-brain.html

• UNCAGING THE HEART

While lying in the bath, or propped up in bed, first do heart breathing of worthiness down into the spleen (left) side of the belly. Then do heart breathing of gratitude down into the liver (right) side of the belly. Use your hands as jumper cables on the heart and the belly to facilitate the energetic shift. Then put your hands on your chest with fingertips meeting at the sternum. Feel into the pressure or cage of the heart and breath into the tension repeating silently "harmony" and "release." After 10 minutes or so of focused frequency change you should have several large spontaneous breaths after which the painful contraction around the heart should let go giving you more space in your chest and freedom to be.

• HEALING THE HEART HOLE

This is a very direct way of addressing pain and deficiency in the heart. You just turn your etheric field from your brainstem back into the heart area at the back of your chest. With the mind's eye imagine lines of magnetic force turning out of your brainstem and looping down into the back of your heart. This works rapidly and is amplified when done during long walks in nature. It can probably used in panic and emotional trauma situations especially if assisted or encouraged by a stable heartfield practitioner.

• TENSION OFF THE HEART

To remove emotional dis-ease from the body requires something like running up and down stairs to really push the heart to blast through "heart ache." The key to social adaptability in providing the energetic stability needed for sovereignty, is to take the tension off of the heart. In this way the Heart is encouraged toward continual opening, rather than contracting and closing in anxiety and fear, which lead to neurosis, exclusion and low Self-love. De-stressing is essential to growth. Huffing Out Breath, Running, Cardio Muscular Release, Jumping Jacks, Boxing and Arm Shaking.

• HEART WINGS MEDITATION

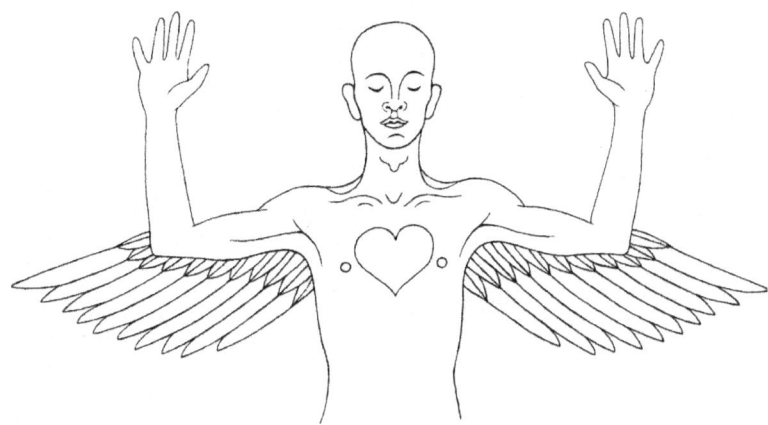

The Heart Wings Meditation is one of the most important Inner Art for getting to the oppressive core of our suffering from shame, fear of rejection and the need to be assimilated (fit in). Lie on your back on the grass with your bare feet facing the sun, and hands raised above your head as though it was a stick-up. Obviously the less clothes you have on the better, but nudity is not necessary. Do the Inner Candle (tongue drop, inner smile, jaw is a dish, central candle through the head, closed eyes up looking at the flame). Breathe into the belly extending the in-breath so that it fills up the very top of the lungs. As you inflate the top of the lungs the upper chest will radiate lines of horizontal force that feel like the wings of a white swan or dove.

Now imagine the in-breath being pulled into a red heart in the center of your chest as you breathe up high to establish the heart's wings. Do no more than 10 breaths the first time you try this because it is a radical workout to the mid back area and so you may need to tap your adrenal-kidney area afterwards. This exercise is perfect for getting rid of the sludge and drudge of Borg repression that gums up the Gate of Life (12th Thoracic), and cages the heart, thereby preventing full vitalizing breath. The Heart Wings Meditation is one of the very best Inner Arts for kick starting autonomic self-regulation, and is an all-round lifesaver when persecuted by the Borg's power tripping.

The combination of the Heartwings Meditation and the Feeding the Roots meditation are companions for profound grounding, after which the dysfunctional complexities are somewhat irrelevant. If you drop the muscles at the back of the tongue and put on an inner smile and tone with the breath to get a good chest resonance going, this will open up your chest more to give your heart room to breath. My sense is that your body might be holding your heart down, because this world is "not really to receive the big you." Be the big you anyway, this will create a life large enough to hold all of you. We are all blind masochists until someone loves us enough to allow us to be our big self. So we must start the process by loving ourselves, this allows others to love their self also.

• HEART BUTTERFLY MEDITATION

Self compassion reduces PTSD and lowers pain, and helps overcome the addictions we use to avoid self-responsibility and self-actualization. Self-love and self-compassion is one of the hardest emotions to generate for those who were alienated, misunderstood and unloved (in a sovereign, not codependent way). Self love in my experience often is only generated when we are under attack and are forced to finally stand up for ourselves and resist abuse. While lying on your back on your bed or on the grass, on the sternum/thymus lock the thumbs together touching at the clavicle to create the butterfly over the breasts. With opposing hands spread over the breasts like butterfly wings. Meditate radiating self-compassion from the heart in association with the breath. Only with the love we generate through ourselves can we then use to love others. If we are hardened against our own existence and suffering, then we are hardened against the world.

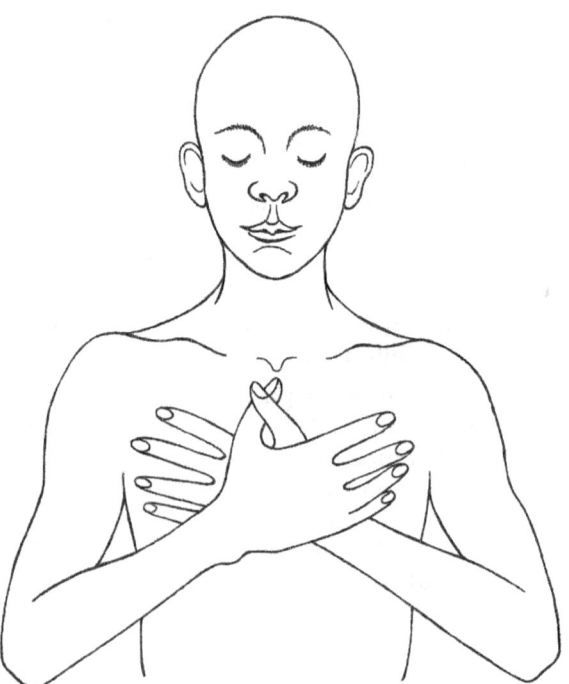

• GROWING SPIRITUAL WINGS

The Inner Arts for releasing the shoulder girdle include: Healing the Heart Hole, Primal Release Pose, Cardio Muscular Release, Upright Walking, Arm Shaking Release and the Spinal Shower. Other exercises to open the wing area for spiritual embodiment include Kunlun, pilates, the wood chopping exercise, boxing and martial arm movements, pressing arms against a door frame, push ups, pull ups, simulated bird-flight and hugging. More methods to release the shoulder girdle include broomstick stretching, rolling on tennis balls, foam rollers, large exercise balls, and shoulder-stands against a wall, plus stretches and twists while hanging inverted. Life is free, release it!

• THE HEARTFIELD EFFECT

Research at the Institute of HeartMath (heartmath.org) shows that heart's magnetic field is approximately 5000 times stronger than the brain's magnetic field and can be detected several feet away from the body with sensitive magnetometers. During sustained feelings of love or gratitude, the blood pressure and respiratory rhythms, among other oscillatory systems, entrain to the heart's rhythm. While negative emotions, such as anger or frustration, are associated with an erratic, disordered, incoherent pattern in the heart's rhythms.

The heart's field acts as a global carrier wave that signals, synchronizes and coordinates psychophysiological processes throughout the body, as pulsing waves of energy radiate out from the heart. Thus the heart acts to inform and in-form the integration of bodily functions as a whole, plus the heart's field is directly involved in intuitive perception, through its quantum relationship to Zeropoint energy for the heart is a quantum capacitor.

Phase-locking or coherence of the heartfield optimizes emotional stability, mental function, and will through enhancing consciousness, sensory awareness and physiological function. Heart coherence influences the heart fields and brain states of those around us, plus the heart acts like an antenna that communicates with the electromagnetic fields produced by the hearts of other individuals. When the communal heartfield is harmonious order, sanity, morality and flow are optimized, which enhances health, psychosocial well-being, and intentional action in the individual or social group. Through the intentional coherence of the communal heart field a shift to planetary transpersonal consciousness can occur that brings humanity into harmony with the wellbeing of the whole.

The heart is a *magnometer* that can sense the gravitics, density, coherency, aliveness, light and emotional state of objects and living things. During kundalini awakenings one my notice a magnetic phenomena of motion towards the electromagnetic axis of the heart at the shoulders. The heartfield is so powerful that during heart expansions objects placed on the chest will flip by perpetual motion towards the right or left shoulder. The atomic heat given off by the heart during expansion phase must be the hotest possible by organic flesh short of spontaneous combustion.

The Alpha brainwave state is considered the brain's most normal functioning state. 8Hz Alpha gives you access to the heart-brain and enteric-brain through the right-hemisphere, and 40Hz Gamma is the wholebrain integrating frequency.

• ARM SHAKING RELEASE

This arm shaking exercise I received in a dream, which showed me how to unlock frozen back muscles associated with a depressed heart function. The Arm Shaking Release activates the rhomboid area between the shoulder blades and opens the Heart center. It acts to warm up the social wiring connected to the arms and relieves tension and grief from the heart and lungs. But it also warms and enlivens the body and releases sadness and morbidity generated from an unsatisfactory social life. By "shaking up" the social wiring we become more liberated, extraverted and interested in the world around us. With feet about one foot apart extend arms downward and slightly forward, shake the shoulders rapidly up and down (pumping not waving). Then isometrically press hands firmly together in front of you with arms still extended downward while breathing deeply.

• HEART DYSAUTONOMIA

The expanded heartfield is hungry for grounding into the earth herself, because we are generally *unpolarized* from being electromagnetically separated from nature's energies. The heart is harmonized by earthing through going barefoot, plus devotional sungazing. Drop the muscles at the back of your tongue and put on the inner smile, this will center you more in your belly and right-brain which takes the pressure off the heart. Remineralizing and re-enzyming with sprouts will allow the heart to gain greater regularity and strength. Fenugreek sprouts have a powerful regulatory effect on the lipid levels in the blood and for conditions that affect cardiovascular health.

• HIGH BLOOD PRESSURE

Hypertension can also lead to other conditions such as congestive heart failure, kidney disease, and blindness. When pressure rises with big weather symptoms or excess energy in the head—Lie in an Epsom salts bath for an hour, drinking 2 pints of water, do the Inner Smile, drop the back of the tongue, tone HUUU, one hand on heart the other on solar plexus and breathe into the solar plexus, and meditate. Finish the bath only after you have urinated 3 times. Anthocyanins, the purple pigments from fruits and vegetables lowers blood pressure. Lecithin helps lower blood pressure in some people by providing choline, a building block for Acetylcholine which is the parasympathetic nervous systems primary neurotransmitter. Taurine, a sulfur aminoacid, lowers blood pressure since it functions as a generalized inhibitory neurotransmitter.

If you feel your nervous system is too sympathetically activated (eg: palpitations, heat, sweating, tingles, high blood pressure etc...) then put some Kava kava, Caapi, Rhodiola, Valerian leaf, Chamomile, Kudzu, Raspberry leaf, Moringa, Ashwagandha, Cat's Claw, Shatavari (*Asparagus racemosus*) and Gota kola into your smoothie base mixture. Other anti-hypertensives include Buchu tea, teas of Red clover and Nettle; Garlic, Celery, Basil, Coleus forskohlii, Lavender, Ginger, Chinese Hawthorn, Mistletoe, Cinnamon, Pomegranate, Taurine and Magnesium citrate.

These dietary and herbal sources are generally more effective at lowering blood pressure than medical drugs, without the side effects. Again, lying on the grass and hanging out in negative ion environments like near waterfalls and moving water will reduce blood pressure and inflammation. The Three Kings Inner Art and long heavy out-breathing are a quick easy fix to stress.

CHAPTER 9

GROUNDING

Civilization should be set upright on its spiritual roots first as the "primary" focus for survival and recovery of the planet and the species.

The earth herself is negatively charged and the atmosphere around us is positively charged. When the negatively charged electrons are transferred between molecules, we call the process oxidation or "rust." The earth's surface is the greatest antioxidant as it is a reservoir for electrons that provide the negative charge, which prevents oxidation. All disease conditions are associated with having an excess positive charge in our body, meaning there is a lack of electrons, or negative charge. An excess positive charge creates an acid pH and oxidation or rust, that is free radical damage from the stealing of electrons. Earthing or being grounded means walking barefoot on the earth or touching the earth someway with our bare skin.

When we are disconnected from the earth's natural negative charge reservoir we are more subject to oxidation, inflammation, aging, degenerative disease and depression. Chronic pain is associated with an imbalance towards excessively positive charged acid condition. Plus problems with mineralization of bones, dental plaque and tooth decay are related to not being grounded. The structure and metabolic function of the body loses intelligence when cut off from contact with Nature's creatrix energy. Only in the past few generations have humans separated themselves from direct physical contact with the earth by wearing synthetic soled shoes and living in homes that elevate the body above the earth.

Shoes, cars, houses, concrete, unnatural fiber clothing, furniture — in fact most of modern life cuts us off from the source of electrons needed to reduce the electromagnetic fallout of Borg culture, with its anti-Phi technology. Pathogens and parasites thrive on us when we are not grounded. Pathogens and cancer loves an acid, electrically imbalanced, ungrounded body, because the immune system cannot protect a cosmically divorced, electrically depolarized, discombobulated and ungrounded body.

Restoring the body's electrical balance by being grounded may be the most significant contribution to vibrant health period! For we have neither the electrons to quench free radicals, nor the energy to feed our electromagnetic field without bare skin contact with the living earth. The closer you are connected directly to the earth via the bare skin, the longer you will live and the less inflammation and disease you will suffer from. The grounding effect of walking or lying on the earth naked changes our respiration rate and immediately detoxifies us, restores alkalinity normalizing our pH, making us relax. The fountain of youth is the earth herself!

Electromagnetic Fields or EMF's are the radio waves that are emitted appliances and wireless devices such as cell phones and computers. By not taking into account EMF effects and earth-biological energies modern technology, housing and clothing has had a catastrophic effect on the health of the human bodymind and society. Whenever we jump into a body of water, like a river or a stream or a lake, or if we walk barefoot in the rain, we are instantly grounded. If you touch a tree, you are grounded…if you touch a metal pole that is stuck in the earth, you are grounded. When you are grounded, you are more resistant to EMF fields, because the EMF hits you and goes right into the ground. The loss of natural grounding allows EMFs and static electricity to interfere with and stress the body's normal bioelectricity, which interferes with health and sleep. Excess stimulation of the nervous system with unnatural weak electric currents interferes with the bio-electrical communications between cells. When bio-electrical communications from nerves are interfered with muscles become tense and remain tight, leading to fatigue, skeletal problems, pain and reduced cognitive efficiency.

Lack of grounding and the consequent electrical stress contributes to degenerative disease and dysregulation of the nervous system, emotions and immune system. Neurons lacking natural environmental and sensory input are hungry for it and tend to over-respond. Going barefoot in nature provides peripheral mechanical afferance or incoming information and the intake of negative ions from the earth. No part of your body gives your brain more input than your feet! Grounding on mother earth with bare feet is essential to maintain electrical balance and micro-circulations of the body, and thus its flows and rhythms. We have greater communion with our Soul when we are barefoot in nature because we loose the excess positive ions associated with acidity and stress, and so our energy becomes more "ordered" or coherent.

The body defends against excess acidity by withdrawing the calcium and magnesium from bones. The Heart needs direct contact with the earth's energy in order to function correctly and to open in love. Grounding in combination with sunlight on the skin reduces the build up of calcium and fatty plaques, and less cardiovascular disease reduces the incidence of dementia in old age. Earth energy is also necessary to mineralize the body, thus we lose the integrity of our physical and EMF structure when ungrounded.

Earthing lowers free radicals, reduces inflammation, raises thyroid function, balances hormones, normalizes cortisol and regulates circadian rhythms. It normalizes cell polarity, increases skin conductance, increases cell membrane charge, raises zeta potential or colloidal capacity, raises blood oxygen levels, improves breathing, prevents blood cell clumping, lowers calcium plaque build up, increases immune cell function, and reduces tendency of excessive rumination over minutiae. Thus we see that health is the default position and to become whole all we need do is remove the artifices of culture that separate us from nature's vital flows. Grounding is essential to love, sanity and the clear perception of Reality. Grounding along with breathing draws off negative-energies and stress bringing order to chaos, helps dissolve fixed patterns and promotes the absorption of new ideas, increases flexibility and confidence, dissolves illusions and heightens intuitive powers.

Lack of grounding is associated with stress, high cortisol, irritability, hypervigilance and paranoia as there is increased free radical oxidation and inflammation occurring. This molecular dissonance disconnects us from the clear reception of our Soul or morphogenic field and with lowered biophoton flow we slip into more negative lower energy states. Touching ground after traveling in cars and planes recalibrates our circadian rhythms restores cortisol levels, and car sickness and jet lag goes away. Going barefoot and grounding helps us overcome cosmic separation, loneliness, loss of spiritual coherency, reduces brain fog, enhances the immune system, reduces sleep problems, turns back the clock on aging and is essentially the fountain of youth. Rooting the Tree of Life provides the stability and will to live by which we can flower as spiritual beings.

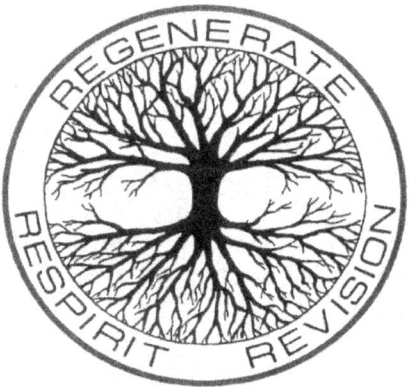

"The Stone, arises from the earth and descends from heaven; thus it gathers to itself the strength of all things above and all things below. Thus when you have the Philosophers Stone, the light of lights, the darkness of ignorance will flee away from you." Emerald Tablet

When a cathode ray from the sun hits an anode of the earth free electrons are liberated from the anode's surface. When we live by Phi and the Tao… that is the way of Nature…we embody more coherent light. As long as light is synotronic and coherent our cells can embody an infinite amount of light, but if our atomic matrix is mal-structured and weak we will leak light until we die from energy loss, oxidation, inflammation and dehydration. The more unobstructed, conductive and electrically alive your body, the more efficient is your grounding, hence the importance of mineral rich raw juices and green smoothies that help to up your zeta potential and cell voltage will also help you to ground. When we detoxify acid toxins, raise our antioxidants, remineralize, re-enzymize, eat raw-remineralized food, reduce cellular inflammation, dearmor, relax internal tension and halt conflicting thought we align the electromagnetic forces of our atoms and molecules such that they spin without destabilization and loss of photons. Thus less light is lost in scattered diffusion and interference, and more biophoton light is condensed within the crystal of our body to power our metabolism and consciousness.

When activated by pressure and movement, nerve endings in the feet called proprioceptors send signals to the brain telling it how the body is oriented. Shoes block these receptors from doing their job and therefore inhibit the development of strong neurological pathways and connections. Proprioceptor stimulation from walking barefoot on uneven terrain creates neuromuscular strength, spacial orientation, balance, and coordination. Science tells us it takes at least 80 minutes of lying on the ground to recharge the blood to the correct polarity so that it doesn't clump. This is a poor substitution for creating a life-supporting, high-biogenic electromagnetic environment in which to earth by every means possible. The ultimate grounding lifestyle is to live somewhere where you can go barefoot. However a good place to start is with the Universal mat, which you can sit on, use under your feet at the computer etc... Grounding the houseplants in your house with copper wires into the earth outside, assists in grounding you by the field effect. The door to returning to the Garden is to "not denature nature" thereby supporting the underlying harmony, integrity and grace prior to dissonance and separation.

TOUCH GROUND

When in a disconnected state we have lost touch with ground control. An organism is only healthy (whole) by being connected to the planet and sky. Earthing supplies electrons cells needed for countering free radicals, reducing acids, the electron chain in ATP production, run the cell membrane pumps and maintaining zeta potential (that is avoiding flocculation and coagulation of body fluids and the clumping of blood cells). Earthing establishes the micro current movements of the water molecules in creating the helical structures of our DNA, proteins and enzymes. With a strong electromagnetic structure our molecules are less likely to mutate, glycate or oxidate. If we are not connected to earth and sky the nano machinery of our molecules cannot engineer themselves into the ideal form for efficient functioning and so we fail to obtain health, wholeness or enlightenment.

As we start to improve the cosmic connection...things line up...and we establish the synergy of wholeness by which humanity could advance geometrically. The key to reorganizing or "wholing" the bodymind from any disease, disorder or distress is the vertical line of the body between earth and sky, and the body's resilience to the pull of gravity. The more grounded and erect the posture, the greater the flow electromagnetic juice and oxygen to the brain, generating the spiritual Presence that vitalizes life and prevents the armoring, shutting down and stunting of growth that prevents us from claiming our full humanity. The higher the cell voltage, the more anti-gravity power the body possesses. During a kundalini awakening there are periods when the light lumination of the body is so great that we get the sense that we are lighter. In fact it is said that well trained monks can even levitate.

By allowing our mass to respond freely to gravity without holding on in stress and contraction, we allow the hexagonal water body to crystallize in perfect Phi. Thus by dropping our mass into the center of the earth we incarnate the spiritual, light or etheric bodymind. For the body's water to flow towards the gravitational center of the earth in perfect Phi we must be physically grounded on nature's earth. The natural flow of water towards the center of the earth regenerates the water's life-giving force. The root or seed form of the vortices in the sacred geometric vortexijah of the HUman body emanates from the core of the earth, thus our relationship to the gravitational neutral centerpoint determines the alignment and attunement of our form and function. This gravitic magnetio-attraction also dictates our capacity for wisdom, for the implosive conjunction of the winding our spin is what allows us to tap into the universal mind-force. This is why meditating and sungazing on iron-rich vertical rocks at sunrise or sunset is one of the finest forms of quickening to initiate kundalini awakening. By sitting on a earth energy conductor under the rays of the sun we marry the heaven and earth, and the father and mother within our atoms. Loving ourselves is the inner alchemy of heaven (Void) and earth (matter) through responding to the magnetic attraction of Spirit.

The levels of consciousness achieved through earth-core grounding, and rock meditation include nonlocal, transtemporal, multiplex vision, global navigation, Psi and remote viewing, Samadhi (unity), transcendental-visionary and active compassion. Once we free ourselves up to respond to the great cosmic winding and music of the spheres on this level, increasingly we become aligned with a higher order of synchronicity, which expands the novelty factor in our experience of happenstance. All knowledge is unfolded from the Void through which we can manifest to our will, should our will be for the universal good. In a way, we were born from the Void, and our life is a return journey to the center from which we began.

Nassim Haramein says the proton is the medium of nonlocal or omniscient consciousness, and Tesla said the hydrogen atom gets its energy from the Void. Thus we have begun to think that it is the body's water, or rather the hydrogen bonding of our living water molecules, that is the telegraphic correspondent of the Vril, Ether, Zeropoint, Brahman or God aspect, as well as the 3D physical realm that our 5 senses can readily perceive. Thus our metabolism has a direct relationship to the formative forces associated with our relationship to the center of the Earth—the Halls of Amenti. (Emerald Tablet on youtube.)

In the youtube video *"The Role of Water in the Electric Body"* Gerald Pollack points to the healing properties of water, air, earth and sun when used in combination for Inner Arts. The sunlight splits water and creates charge by charge separation. Light increases the viscosity of water, thereby increasing work done such as detoxification, energy generation (respiration) and cell nutrition, not to mention elemental transmutation. Read about this in *"Cells, Gels and the Engine of Cells,"* by Gerald Pollack.

The health of the sovereign body brings out the health of others. There is no avoiding the reality of the embodiment of spirit and flow of Chi energy. The art of right conduct and successful living arises from our relationship to heaven and earth, in the bodymind's degree of electrical conductivity. If we are not rooted into the earth then we are not tapping into the **Zeropoint Field**, consequently we are not rooted into our Sou's Muse, nor do we have an intact fulcrum for balanced exchange and reciprocity in relationship.

Trying to heal or become whole when we are separated from the great mother and father principle is like trying to swim in the air. This brings to question our entire cultural behavior of building concrete cities, wearing shoes and sunglasses, living and working in buildings and wearing plastic clothing. In separating ourselves from the electric earth, we become a parasite for we cannot conduct right, nor engage in right conduct. On the nature of sacred cosmology see: John Worrell Keely, Walter Russell and Viktor Schauberger, Ananda Bosman, Dan Winter, Marko Rodin, David LaPointe and Nassim Haramein.

• ROOTING INTO THE EARTH

Personal power is achieved by grounding and rooting deeply into the earth's energies, a process that helps the body to earth via its root chakra, the spine and the feet. The primary grounding method is to walk or run barefoot on the bare earth or to lie your spine on the earth for at least half an hour a day, while feeling the pull of gravity. Hang out by a spring, stream or waterfall while you do this and you get bonus points. Living water relaxed through gravity and earth energies, as found in deep spring water, is the premium water for cellular hydration, and for maintaining the structural integrity of proteins, DNA and other biomolecules, for energizing the body, empowering innate healing and enhancing toxin removal from cells. Wearing grounding stones like Hematite or Red Garnet.

The Spinal Shower is a great way to for remove extra static energy from the nerves and tissues. Grounding exercises include lying on one's back and forcefully pushing one's feet against a wall or tree. Dancing is good for increasing energy conduction. Native American type foot stomping dances build up the piezoelectric conductivity of the leg bones and strengthen the nerves making the legs better conductors of earth energy. Standing in the Maori Haka position, which is kind of like a gorilla stance and stamping one leg at a time, actually doing the facial expressions, vocals, hand and feet movements is a big bonus—see Haka videos on youtube. Put some more green plants around your computer, and a negative ion generator for your computer room or an indoor waterfall.

Of course there are the traditional methods of grounding, horse riding, pottery making, gardening or farming. Walk more rather than driving around in cars and spend more time outside of buildings. Move to Hawaii or vacation there, it's the primary grounding location on the planet. Meditate at sunrise or sunset on iron rich rocks. Lie on the ground at night looking at the stars. Hug a tree, or go to sleep under trees. Need I say that sex will help reduce extra brain electric interference, but it may also increase kundalini. Any kind of body-work, swims or water therapy. A clay body pack or mud bath will remove excess positively charged ions. If you have synthetic carpet in your home it might be best to replace it with something more natural, either a wool carpet, or wood or bamboo. Being around animals, pets and children is also grounding.

> *The untold wealth of unconditionally loving one's own heart regardless of circumstances is discovered only on the inside.*

• FEEDING THE ROOTS

To become "whole" we must find the upper limit of resonance by growing our spiritual roots into the earth by sending an bioelectromagnetic wave through the ground to pass through the iron core of the earth. Lie face down on the grass in the sun, hands up by your head in stick-up position with palms down. Drop your body into the earth, and when you have made contact, then with your whole being send an electrical charge with your breath down into the earth. With each deep breath send another radiant charge into the earth. When the wave reaches the far side of the planet, it bounces back, it returns to the point of origin. Then if we send out another charge with the next breath the two will combine, go out, and bounce again, reinforcing the initial pulse and the wave builds up power. In this way we can use the entire planet as a conductor and transformer by sending successive pulses through it, modifying the ground's electrical potential and changing it from an electrical sinkhole to an electrical source in interrelationship, or sympathetic resonance to us. Restoring our rapport, affinity, compatibility, empathy, groove, togetherness and unity with the earth, and so making contact with our cosmic Being, Christ or soul. Active Grounding connects us to our spiritual roots to promote vital new growth.

• ACTIVE GROUNDING

Apparently thinking, focusing, felt-sensing and visualizing radiant light in the brain or any other part of the body increases photon emissions in that area. We are like a light bulb that we can turn on at will to radiate to infinity, and so connect to the All. In the Inner Arts exercises we start off by establishing the felt sense of the inner structure we are connecting to and then we light it up and make it radiant. This "turning on the switch" to energy flow generates more light energy to flow. That is, in a commodified culture we become increasingly alienated, deprived and dispossessed no matter how many material goods we acquire, because we tend to stop short at the material surface of things, while not establishing a loving felt-sense connection with the world around us. Thus we remain cut-out-figures of our true radiant being would not afraid to feel into and engage its environment.

To rectify this disconnected state, with the Inner Arts we actively turn on the juice and pour light from our body. We then find that only by "radiating" can we come fully alive and fulfilled. Our reality is animated by what we ourselves put into it. If we remain mechanical and mere a stick figure of our true Self we will live a life of gnawing dissatisfaction, dissonance and insufficiency. We live lives of quiet desperation and fear simply because we have not yet learnt how to "turn on the juice." You are what you radiate! When it comes to energy exchange, what we put out is what we get back…plus much more.

Radiating and building the strength of our ability as a quantum capacitor becomes a need more primary and immediate than food. In fact you could say that radiating connective fire (Chi, Light, Blue Flame, Scalar waves) is the greatest food there is. I have found that grounding is not just a process of sucking up earth energy, but of radiating energy into the Axis Mundi, which greatly amplifies the restorative effect by reconnecting us to matter and spirit. It pays to remember we can only go up in Spirit as far as we can go down into Matter, for consciousness is perceived through the instrument of the crystalline frequency receiver of the body.

The reason the Inner Arts are ideally done outside is because lying on the ground removes the static, as well as providing the body with electrons for antioxidation and reducing inflammation. Inflammation (or free radical oxidation) is one of the major sources of inefficiency, incoherence and disorder in the bodymind, thus a significant cause of our unenlightenment, aging and decrepitude. The Inner Arts should always be used in association with grounding on the earth and natural light wherever possible to help establish higher homeostasis. If you are already depleted you will need to be using nature's energies to augment your own—even as you "normalize" yourself. Thus sungaze, lie on the ground daily, do your Inner Arts by a stream or under the stars, swim in the ocean, run in meadows, sit under a waterfall etc... It is very hard to pull yourself up by your bootstraps when you do not have any boots, and nature is always the foundation and source of our healing.

I got the idea for **active or radiant grounding** from Tesla's experiment with the aerial apparatus for the utilization of radiant energy www.electroherbalism.com/Bioelectronics/Tesla/Tesla_greatest_hacker.htm

• PERSONAL GROUNDING DEVISES

The Earth's mass is an electrolytic conductor on the bioelectrical environment of the human organism. What grounding does is to instantly drain off excess positive charge, induced voltage from EMF toxicity and ion imbalance, thereby allowing the body to operate with less "noise" in its bioenergy circuits and signaling mechanisms. The Earth's electromagnetohydrodynamic potential plays a fundamental role in regulation of bioelectrical and bioenergetical processes. Contact to the earth by a copper conductor with a moistened surface of the human body evokes a rapid decrease of electrostatic potential on the body and in venous blood to the value of approximately −200 mV. This confirms the idea of using a copper grounding wire and wrist attachments of other terminals applied to the body during Inner Arts in outside environments such as on the grass. I am also in favor of creating outside offices for computer work and writing in which the feet are grounding into the earth through copper rods, copper wires and copper ankle bands.

Copper grounding rods with copper wrist bands can be used for geomantic charging while doing spiritual and healing sessions on the grass. Grounding rods for connecting up the body during meditative yoga like the Inner Arts can give us a **-200mV** charge which can reduce the time it takes for the blood and tissues to recharge themselves. Ultimately I am going to live in a house with a polished hempcrete floor that contains magnetite sand and volcanic ash in the hempcrete and that incorporates a grid of copper grounding rods.

Unless we are super rich or super poor we are not likely to live in a clay floor strawbale house anytime soon. Thus we must work with what we have by incorporating grounding mats, earthing sheets, grounding shoes and going barefoot, lying on the grass, earthen furniture, sleeping outside, and getting into subtle energy devises such as radionics, orgonite, pyramid structures, geomancy, paramagnetics, magnetic therapy, light and sound frequencies, crystals, essential oils, ORMUS, structured water, negative ions, plant energies, sacred geometry architecture, and natural fiber clothing. To counter toxic frequencies diet should be largely raw and must include high antioxidants and plentiful colorful pigments, along with olive leaf and plentiful greens, microgreens and sprouts. Grounding, magnetite sand foot baths, grounding shoes, earthen floored houses, basalt floors, negative ion generators, indoor fountains, houseplants and EMF protection will become ever more important. Crystals, orgonite devices, shungite pendants, radionic devices should be employed.

"The deeper you go in connecting the more autonomous you become within yourself and if you are not autonomous within yourself, then there is nothing THERE to connect with anything else." Sten Linnander greenplanetfm.com

• ISOMETRIC STRETCHES

Isometric means "equal" and "length." These exercises are performed without altering the length of muscles. To assimilate kundalini some strengthening integrating exercises might be in order. The upper-body wall press is perhaps the perfect exercise for integrating heart expansions. I found that when the autonomic White Shock made me "not in my body," then leg presses against the wall helped me to come back into my body. Pushing into a wall or against a doorframe with the arms and legs and hanging by the finger tips from the top of a door frame is similarly helpful.

When performing repetitive, rhythmic movements such as Isometrics, Qigong or yoga the cerebellum triggers activity within the frontal lobes that then signals the nucleus acumens to release dopamine and endorphins, similar to "runner's high," which gives us a sense of greater embodiment and empowerment. **Habituation** occurs within the cerebellum by performing repetitive, rhythmic movements. It takes approximately twenty minutes of movement to induce habituation in untrained individuals and less than ten minutes of movement. The habituation response triggers activity within the frontal lobes that then signal the nucleus acumens to release dopamine and endorphins.

The release of these hormones is associated with "runner's high." Unlike the runners high, the dopamine produced during a Qigong-induced habitation response, is released in an environment free of physiological stress, oxygen deprivation and cortisol stress hormones. This peaceful environment is conducive to the absorption of dopamine., encouraging the brain to continue this balancing activity. At this point we add vibro-acoustic toning to vibrate the skull, cleaning cerebral spinal fluid, enabling better transmission of neural transmitters across the synaptic gaps and enhancing re-uptake of those hormones. Vibro-acoustic tones vibrate the sphenoid bone, the sternum and stimulates the pituitary's release of hormones.

• WAR HAKA

The ultimate movement practice for emotional strength and grounding is the Maori Haka. The Haka is a Maori war dance that precedes battle, in order to motivate the warriors psychologically and to unbalance and terrorize the enemy. It is delivered with loud shouting and forceful flexing arm movements, to invoke the god of war and to discourage and frighten the enemy. It involves fierce facial expressions and grimaces, poking out of the tongue, eye bulging, grunts and cries, waving of weapons and rhythmic thumping of the thighs, biceps and chest. The hands, arms, legs, feet, voice, eyes, tongue and the body as a whole combine to express courage, annoyance or aggression. The haka is an excellent kundalini tool, both for raising kundalini, freeing its movement and for grounding and integrating the energy. It will also enhance confidence and improve the immune, lymphatic and circulation systems and clear the lungs. Also will also eliminated stagnant energy from the nervous system and aids in the liberation of pent-up or repressed emotions. There are plenty of version of the Haka on web videos.

• HAMSTRING STRETCH

This hamstring stretch is life changing as it releases vast amounts of energy. It not only feels good to stretch this commonly tight area, but hamstring flexibility is also important for the health of your back, hips, and knees.

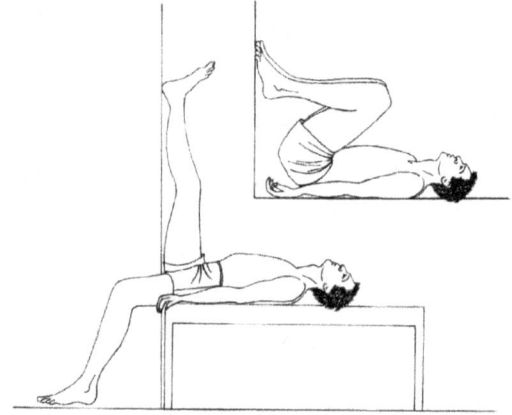

This delicious hamstring stretch can be done at home or at a destination in your locale that you run to. It is good to do the second one on the grass with your legs pushing into a tree to loosen up the sacrum at the bottom of the spine. Most knee problems are created due also to the tightening of the hamstrings. Lengthening the hamstrings will help enormously by providing space within the knee joint. This is no easy matter, the hamstrings are very fibrous and resist stretching. These postures even have a grounding effect for those whose hips, hamstrings, and spine present resistance to the light.

Fascia is the primary energy conductor of the body, receiving electrons, from the surface of the earth, which are powerful antioxidants. The fascia in the back of the legs once contracted prevents energy from the ground rising through the body. Unblocking, relaxation and softening comes from letting go of tension, which allows the entire body-field to become more illuminated. In fact, you may not be aware of how much tension you have until you let it go. Flexibility exercises should be relaxing. Avoid over-stretching. Never stretch to the point of pain or discomfort. Always stretch slowly and evenly and don't forget to breathe.

• ACUMASSAGE RUNNING

It is interesting to run barefeet with a relaxed foot-rolling gate with the center of gravity on the point between acupuncture points Kidney 1 and Kidney 2. It is energizing, effortless and post mechanical (post egoic). Extend the foot rolling relaxed gait up the spine so that you feel like a jelly gorilla. Focus on fully oxygenating your workout and feeling into the body's movements. Acussage Running on grass or the beach greatly enhances the benefits.

• THE ASS PUSH UP

For the Core Lower Body this interesting strengthening stretch hits the legs, buttocks and lower back, as well as massaging and loosening the spine.

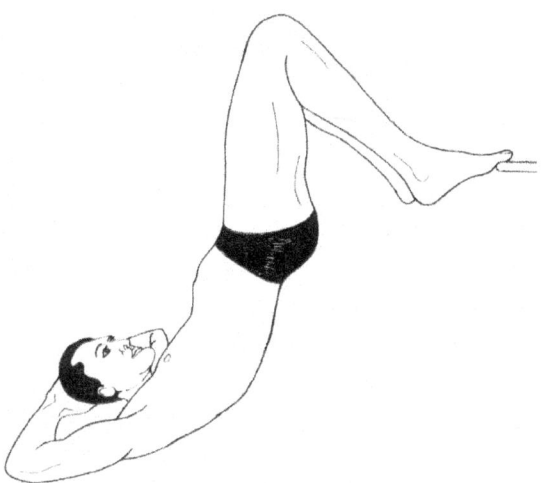

Lie on your back on the floor beside a desk or table (height of which depends on your leg length). Hands on the floor interlocked behind the head. Push your feet against the lip of the desk and raise your buttocks high as you can off the floor, extending the back stretch into the rhomboid area. Push up and hold the upward stretch for a deepening of the effect. Repeat as many times as you like. This is also excellent for working the abdominal region and the lymphatics.

• ANIMAL YOGA

The ultimate gym or yoga studio is in nature. To reinstate our connection with the planet and the deeper parts of ourselves this practice of animal yoga is done in natural environments…in your back yard, a park or wilderness. First ground the body by lying on the grass on your back, front and sides for a while. Then using the nature around you—the grass, the trees, the rocks—put yourself into various animal postures while feel-sensing yourself as that animal. Some possible animals to try are the dog, cat, frog, rabbit, seal, monkey, turtle and bear. Use the full tactile impact of the environment around you to get deeply into the various postures to explore the spirit of the animal. Because it is an attempt to more fully enter the electromagnetic sensorial environment, animal yoga is best done in the nude if possible, in full contact with the natural world around you. That which is indigenous to nature is endowed with natural grace, supports the soul's journey and a beautiful connection to the natural world. What we love, we are able to do well. We can ultimately only succeed in our naturally gifted genius by working in close proximity to nature.

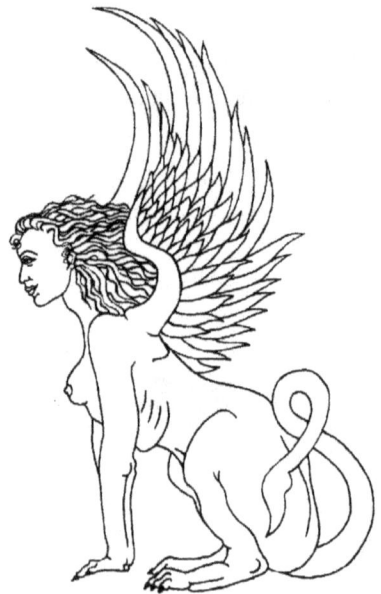

• KUNLUN

Charging Relate-ability—Ideal energy exercises for building relate-ability use the Kunlun idea of holding a big imaginary beach ball while sitting down. Arms are extended and fingers nearly touching out in front of you, while sitting on a chair with feet on the floor. You hold this position for about 5 minutes and then cup the hands over the belly button (hara) for another 5 minutes to generate fire in the belly. It is very enlivening.

You can also do it with hands on the top and bottom of the big ball so that the top hand comes up to about chin height and the bottom is just off the seated legs. After you have done this for a while then you do the same exercises with the heels raised off the ground as well. It is important to do the Inner Smile and conscious breathing during these invigorating exercises to open the Heart chi flow. You can finish of this sequence by putting your hands at the back of your neck with your fingers touching and elbows extended out. Then push your neck gently and firmly back into your hands and hold for several minutes…integrate with hands over hara and breathing. This will strengthen and relax your neck allowing greater energy flow in and out of the head. www.kunlunbliss.com/

The roots of the nervous system are fed by diverting the focus of consciousness away from fear, scarcity and hopelessness, and turning it towards love, abundance and hope. If the roots still abide in impoverished soil then the individual or community cannot rise towards the sun, nor nurture and sustain themselves. The shift towards sovereignty begins when we tend our own soil and turn towards the light of the sun for sustenance. You cannot get to God via mere cognition—the bodymind cannot realize homeostasis or peace without electromagnetically and devotionally replugging into the cosmos. Grounding into the earth and the Cosmos, is a matter of surrender and relaxation…it is prior to the division of the divisive, defensive personality. Thus to be sovereign is to be larger than our known selves.

• KUNDALINI !KUNG DANCE

The Kung are a people living in the Kalahari Desert in Namibia, Botswana and in Angola dance for many hours to "heat" up the n/um (kundalini) so that the !kia state (transcendence) can be attained. This involves the peak experience of going beyond the ordinary self to experience the participation mystique (eternity). Passing through thresholds of fear, kundalini heats up in the pit of the stomach and rises from the base of the spine to the skull where transcendence (Satori) occurs. The !Kung dance all night and raise kundalini by which they perform healing, and all !Kung men are considered healers.

The singing, stomping and autonomic pelvis giggling is essential to getting the spark to rise up the spine. Note the intense grounding and immune stimulation that would come from barefoot dancing. The African tribes dance as a spiritual practice for effect, purpose and meaning—for coherence, coordination, cooperation and plugging to the Gaian mind. They invented trance dance quarter of a million years ago or more. They don't dance for performance, entertainment or appearance but for changes in the state of consciousness and conforming to the evolutionary groove. The Kung use kundalini energy in a sacred ritual to tap psychic information and precognition to enhance the welfare of the tribe. Conditions that contribute to this kind of communal kundalini raising include fasting, music, drumming and a fire around full or new moon.

WETTER WATER

Water is the most solvent of all liquids. If the body's water is acidic, sticky, and toxic it is unable to serve its biological function as the dissolving solute and reactive catalytic medium for metabolic processes. The increase in the viscosity or stickiness of cell protoplasm and body fluids due to cooked and damaged foods is associated with the dehydration, contraction and congestion of tissue. In fact aging and disease is directly related to cellular dehydration, decreased colloidal capacity and decreased viscosity or "flow." Lowering surface tension and increasing the electric conductivity or **zetapotential** helps cells to maintain their EMF shields so that they don't stick together. Positive thoughts and emotions also increase the viscosity of fluids, perhaps by altering pH, hydrogen ions, hydrogen bonding angles and the microwave/light/sound forms in water. Wetter water means more toxins out and more nutrients in.

Rainwater is the most pure and organized water on the planet and absorbs immediately into and hydrates plant, animal and human cells. This water passes through the body but cannot penetrate cells without lower surface tension. In the body, only water with "low surface tension" fully hydrates. In order for toxins to leave the cells and nutrients to enter the cells, the cells must be in contact with water that has a low surface tension. Without low surface tension toxins cannot be removed from cells and the cells die due to accumulation of their own waste products. Dehydrated cells become catabolic, meaning the body starts utilizing its own tissue for energy production, resulting in degeneration of cellular health and immune response.

Cell membranes are phospholipids (fats), which have low surface tension of about 45 dynes/cm. Cells require a surface tension of roughly the same range for water to wet the cells, thus allowing the water to pass through the fatty acid cell wall carrying nutrients and vitamins. Ordinary water has a HIGH surface tension which means it has a difficult time wetting the cells within the body. Normal tap water has a surface tension of 73 dynes/cm, while distilled water is 72 dynes/cm at 25 °C (77 °F), which means that the water is able to move cells through the body, but is not capable of penetrating the cell. However fresh squeezed organic juices get toxins out and nutrients due to their low surface tension.

Just 30 minutes of **solar disinfection** of water, after which lemon juice is added is effective at greatly reducing E. coli levels. Lemon/lime juice is 33 dynes/cm so adding it to water reduces the surface tension of the water making it more hydrating…thereby aiding the lymphatic system and kidneys by clearing out inorganic minerals and the morbid accumulation of acidic toxins. You can add a squeeze of lemon or lime juice to water to lower surface tension as well to make it more alkaline, thereby increasing cellular hydration and detoxification. As we age the depletion of hydrogen in the tissues may lead to many of the symptoms of the aging process. Hydrogen-rich water is antioxidant, anti-aging, boosts metabolism, reduces fatigue and improves mood. As hydrogen is the smallest element in the universe, it easily penetrates the entire body, including the neurons and the cell nuclei. To purchase a Hydrogenizer Bottle with Titanium electrodes to avoid heavy metal poisoning email H2@wingscoaching.com

CHAPTER 10

REGENEROSITY EXERCISES

• GRATITUDE

The increasing sense of being at home and being Alive makes metamorphosis seem inevitable. As the awakening speeds our incarnation, a feeling of objective conscience (*baraka*) and gratitude arises as a powerful urge to go-with this force of evolution. For the spiritual drive of Eros is our own deepest source and condition of being that we share with all Life. If we do not listen and surrender to this feeling of right-will, we will resort to sense gratification and self-destruction in an effort to avoid our Self. Keeping in touch with the inner sun, the Heru, Horus or Hero Within is achieved through the pure felt-sense of gratitude. Gratitude is synonymous with courage that ties us into the All, integrates and makes us whole, and is the measure of our aliveness. Receiving is akin to gratitude, and gratitude is akin to giving in return. Radiating from Source and Gratitude…are one and the same thing. For in that is gratitude that returns through us lovingly to all else in reception of life. Radiant love requires nothing in return, merely to be actually received is enough to build reciprocity.

• BLUE-SKY CLUB

By living with the sense of an infinite up-spiral we join the "Blue-Sky Club." This life-stance involves frictionless creativity where we just open up to Spirit and let it flow without barrier, second-guessing or analysis. In this way we follow our bliss and live our authentic hero's/heroine's journey in co-creating a new world of synthesis, negative entropy or cosmic self-ordering. The up-spiral divine play of the Blue-Sky Club is highly contagious for it reflects the natural exuberant genius and timing of Spirit itself. When we join the Blue-Sky Club we become a **Great Attractor** to the building of the new synergistic culture and seemingly impossible events in the external world magically and synchronistically conspire to come together. As you are doing your up-right walking you will notice that the blue sky features prominently in your upper field of vision. The infinite blue is already there, as an ever present backdrop to the finite focus of one's present journey.

• FREEDOM MEDITATION

We overcome the helpless feeling of encroaching fascism, predation, extortion and usurpation through changing our cellular vibration. You can do this with the use of the tongue drop, inner smile, hands on solar plexus, throaty breath, feeling into your cells and silently repeating freedom. Continue to do this until you feel free, and then test your freedom not in confronting jailers or bullies, but it doing exactly what you want to do.

• SUBSTANTIATION MEDITATION

In order to be Muse focused rather than symptom (personality) focused we need to build up the integrative wiring between the sensorymotor center (cerebellum) and the pilot (prefrontal lobes). Working through the closure, self-hatred, self-criticism and trauma damage, we repair the neurology of neurotic divisiveness and latency by establishing richer dendrites and glia cells in the brain. One exercise for re-integration, which serves to move us out of deprivation consciousness and paradoxical intent, is a meditation of affirmative self-talk for enrichment of the wiring for "potential." Lie down with a cervical pillow under the neck and a bolster under the knees.

Put on a meditation CD similar to Jeffrey Thompson's Gamma (40Hz) with earphones. You can also opt to cover eyes with a buckwheat eye sack and hold onto the copper pipes of a **Hilda Clarke Zapper**. Then with the mind's eye focus your attention into the prefrontal lobes and use simple affirmative language to silently "talk" to your forehead. Such as: You are doing well; You are so good; Allowing; Complete; Joy; You are so sweet; Fullness; Unity; Gratitude; Faith; You are totally free; Anything is possible if I make it happen, etc… Drinking a bunch of water and doing this whole process nude in the sun while lying on the ground would stake more "functions" into the meditation.

• OVERCOMING INERTIA TO CHANGE

The least amount of fragmentation means the greatest amount of structure and order. Intent can be recorded and carried in water memory and the subtle energy fields. To facilitate change both our inner and outer worlds need to be cleansed of energetic pollution to reduce fragmentation and thus perpetuate health/wholeness. The Intention Cycle incorporates purification, energizing, organizing, healing, aligning, surrendering, receiving, protecting, releasing. Momentum for change is generated and sustained by a well integrated daily lifestyle that incorporates both physical, emotional, mental, social and spiritual super-nutrition.

• INNER COSMIC TREE

This is a powerful head-body integrating exercise that makes you feel "substantial," complete and in full integrity/integration (truth). While outside standing barefoot on the earth imagine (feel and envision) yourself as a tree… with branches reaching into your head, and branching out into your chest and roots spreading out into the soil. By holding this sensation you will find that you are centered very strongly in your throat and brainstem. Stand like a tree, arms outstretched, feel your roots going down into the ground. Absorb energy from the sunlight, feel deeply connected to the energies of the cosmos. Feel your natural innate abundance and tacit longing to radiate the beauty of creation. Become!

• WORKING WITH EXCALIBUR, THE SILVER CORD

Stand tall with shoulders back, breathing slow and deep; chin up, stomach pulled in, pelvis tucked under, with feet about a foot apart. Imagine a silver-white lightening rod extending through your spine, shooting up into the sky from the crown of your head, and extending deep into the ground from the coccyx. As you draw energy in to the Silver Cord it begins to glow and pulsate, dispersing energy through your body. By plugging oneself into the cosmos, this lightening rod connecting heaven and earth generates energy that can be used for healing yourself or others.

• VISIONARY TUNE UP

Drink two glasses of water and lie on the grass under a tree. Breathing "appreciation," "harmony," "order," "peace" in through the heart and exhale the quality throughout the body via conscious breath. Focus on something specific to look forward to, something you want to do, and build the image of that up in your mind. As soon as you engage in dreaming up a fun future, your body-mind-spirit will fall into natural coherent clarity. Kundalini will tell you exactly what to do if you listen deeper and deeper, dropping further into the felt-sense of the intelligence of the body's higher wisdom.

• LIVER OPENING

To dance in a field of glory you have to open up and unburden the liver. Put your left hand on the heart, right hand on liver. Breathe in gratitude through your heart, then on the out-breath you silently say gratitude again and push it down into the liver, moving your fingers over the liver to awaken it. Try raw milk thistle porridge, methylators like garlic mustard, Shizandra berry and NAC with Molydenum and Selenium also.

• SOLAR RUB

While lying in bed (or generally throughout the day) rub your solar plexus in a circular motion. Rub it gently until any anxiety or difficulty residing in your solar plexus is gone and you feel "full" and satisfied. Buddha nature is being able to let go of the past and live contented in the present. This is the source of the fountain of spiritual abundance.

• SOURCE CHARGING

Sungaze at dawn or dusk with eyes open…get the feeling that you are becoming filled up with photons from the sun as though you were recharging your batteries, with special focus on your heart. Then close your eyes, and imagine that you are sending loving light out from your pineal gland (third eye), spreading it like a floodlight around the world.

• CHOPPING WOOD

Stand with feet apart, place palms together and bend over chopping your arms between your legs. As you go over in your chop breath out and let out a loud HAH! Sound from the belly. Continue to do this until you contact and release your deep sense of abandonment, deprivation and grief. This is a good exercise to do in healing groups around sex abuse, enslavement and lack of sovereignty.

• EMBRACE THE SERPENT

To create a revolution in evolution we must "release" consciousness from the body armor and overcome the inertial drag of the past, to bring about awakening of full creativity and passion for life. As we wake up we may notice our ego is out of control and we seem to be fighting ourselves, and this is separating us from our "life." Instead of fighting with your ego, simply ask it what it needs. The best place to start with divisiveness and distortion is to work regularly on opening the body armor. To open muscles and detoxify you need more magnesium eg: magnesium citrate and greens. A high enzyme raw diet will provide the fastest transformation. Try a heating pad or hot water bottle on your stomach. Heaps of floor exercises and stretches with a Plastic Roller Ball, yoga, inner arts, breathing and breath-walks will loosen the contraction, oxygenate and raise your operating mode. (Fabrication Enterprises Cando Inflatable Roller for dearmoring via spinal rolling.)

Then when in a high rev organize a special event for your family, say a weekend at hot springs or something. By working to create a higher functioning life filled with love, joy and creativity you will raise your being out of the self-recursive funk, and so the difficulty you now fight with will not even be there anymore. If you stay in your present energy hole you will find endless garbage to deal with and preoccupy you from reaching higher levels of living. You do not have to continue to live in or work through difficulty, if you raise your energy level and clarity to get out of it. Desire governs what one draws forth from the uncreated implicate order and infinite potential.

• FULLNESS PRINCIPLES

Original Blessing, Always Already OK, apriori healing, infinite inner potential, apriori richness, cup overflowing, fecundant resourcefulness, lush wild commons, the wisdom of Nature, thriving creativity cycle, intact and fertile energy and resource cycles from soil to soul, move to get in the groove. That is when we nurture the good and the true the darkness falls away. To maintain the evolutionary continuum we feed the roots to support the shoots. Growth requires that we remove the inhibitions to growth so Self-harm is not an option. We tread the path of fullness by imagining and projecting a clear, positive vision of where we are headed, and a proactive practice in the direction of our vision. Abundance, potency and creativity arise by transforming consciousness at the subconscious, subatomic level, to eliminate limiting belief systems and harness the law of attraction.

• UNCONDITIONAL HAPPINESS

Peace is a condition we generate prior to circumstance. Thus we must go plug into our maker regardless of external conditions or internal story. The more we meditate the more the peace vibe infiltrates our lives. Lie on your back with one leg cocked to the knee of the other (tree pose). Put your hands crossed over your diagram, breathing easy. Drop your mind and generate happiness for no good reason. As you do this as a daily practice, perhaps prior to sleep, you will remember the state of unconditional happiness in your daily life and not get caught up in the drama of egos.

• OVERCOMING ADDICTION TO NOT YET, AND NOT ENOUGH

I am not a big fan of relying on external healers, gurus, spiritual systems or religions. They are for people on threshold of the return to mystic Selfhood. I am more in favor of artists, musicians, enthnobotonists and genuine shamans as psycho-spiritual change agents for they offer genuine food for the development of the whole HUman and the evolution of the soul. Artists who make their living from their art through the expression of spirit are shining examples of sovereigns. We are already whole when we drop our resistance to the cosmic heartbeat, by deeply felt relaxation into the effortlessness, fullness, nectar and satiety of the sovereign or core being.

• THE SOVEREIGN GROUND OF BEING

When we abandon ourselves for someone who's undeserving of our energy, our inner-child is usually hurting deeply and feeling afraid to be alone. Pseudo-leaders, teachers and healers may take people up the garden path for a certain period of time, but ultimately most people eventually want to stand on their own two spiritual feet. The sovereignty meme is the most addictive, empowering, supportive and illustrious meme in the Universe, because it IS the fabric of existence itself. Every moment of our lives the FACT of our cosmic consciousness is steering us in the face. So eventually we all must turn to the ground of our being as our ultimate source of sustenance and knowledge, or remain a insatiable vagrant — a mere consumer of life.

• DIVINE PLAY

The term spirituality has become watered down so I thought of a new term — it is DIVINE PLAY! Divine Play is simply moving out of deprivation consciousness and into the innate abundance and unlimited potential of spirit in each and every moment. *Friedrich Schiller said that Man is not fully human unless he is at play!* Joy is the universal lubricant and perhaps the ultimate integral practice. When paralyzed by your problems and stress, you're unable to deal with life effectively. People who "feel" better make better decisions, think faster on their feet and interact with others in more positive and productive ways. Clear sight (hindsight, foresight, insight, oversight) involves resolving the tension of separation between the self and the world and reconciling division to tacitly know that sovereignty of all life is the fundamental law of the universe. The fallen nature of mankind in its insanity and criminality involves degrees of ignorance of this law. The Inner Arts practice and philosophy is for self-disclosure, self-meeting, self communion and self-development. Bless yourself and all existence, ask for guidance, and don't look for demons, but for daemons.

The way of evolution and transcendence is to redeem the dark by turning it into the light.

CHAPTER 11

SOCIAL META-ADAPTATION

Kundalini cannot be separated from Eros or the Muse for the soul and Kundalini appear to be the SAME THING.

Balancing the neurological development of the "two-faced" Janus (the inner and outer) through the meditative Inner Arts not only affords us a peaceful center within chaotic surroundings, but brightens our faculty of clear seeing the world. Clear seeing from a place of peace means we are not at odds with the world, nor are we undone by it. Inner conflict ends when the inner Janus and the outer Janus are reconciled. It is obviously important to see clearly in order to catalyze transformational change without abusing our new found power or trying too hard to control others and manipulate the change process. The meditative arts reduce the noise to signal ratio, thereby allowing highly coherent spin and the "stillness" of consciousness through which deeper seeing, sensing, feeling, thinking and knowing is possible.

The Inner Arts in a way are a self-processing and also a social composting process. In Hindbrain society the social pressure is to be on top of the pile, in order to avoid suffering the humiliation of being on the bottom. This turns relationships into power allegiances, power conflicts, power dominations, power vampirism, power deceptions and power addictions. By "power" what we really mean is the "freedom to execute our will." Thus anything that increases our ability to execute our will increases our freedom and our power. Consequently relationships in Borg society form around money, property, resources, position, intellect, education, class, breeding, inheritance, talent, genius, sexuality, beauty, personal magnetism, character, humor etc... We form allegiances out of a drive to increase our power in a society that demands we either be powerful or powerless. Negative power uses underhanded, devious, backdoor, dark and destructive methods to get on top.

If you don't go along with the existing rules and symbols of the community's power expectations then you are likely to be marginalized, excluded and prejudiced against, and find it impossible to engage in healthy relationship transactions in a society whose power programs are incompatible with your own level of sensitivity and ethics. Our drive for power in a disempowering society makes us relationship addicts, creates moral deficiency and prevents the realization of sovereign empowerment. Every relationship we enter therefore is a pointer to moving out of the sick power-driven culture and into the healthy love-driven culture. The spiritual suffering caused by relationship addiction is a sign that we have betrayed our Self, lost our core connection and gone off course in an attempt to gain an "external form of power" in order to go along with and comply with the existing power-over paradigm.

We can get back on track by asking ourselves the question: "How can we create the most good?"When the drive for power is taken up by the Hindbrain instead of the Forebrain moral inefficiencies ensue connected to the antilibidinal ego's self-interest at the "expense" of others. The Hindbrain power-drive exhibits negative will, bad faith, scarcity mentality, hording, selfishness, avarice, vanity, arrogance, envy, crime, competition and resource wars. As such an Anti-Golden-Rule is in force that comprises of deliberate malice aforethought and plotting to bring harm and hurt to another. Power-addiction involves enlisting others to bring harm and hurt to another and feeding off the pain of the victim.

Hindbrain injustice involves the projection of "evil out there," in order to create special "in-groups," to justify collective hatred, persecution and exploitation. Power-over is obviously a sin against life as is evident in the emotions it creates in the perpetrator and victim alike, therefore when Hindbrainers enact their power-drive they invariably seek coconspirators and comrades in arms in order to carry out their crimes against life with less of a guilty conscience. Because the Hindbrain's approach to power through the Anti-Golden-Rule is subversive to their spiritual development and emotional health we can only assume that it is a "internal saboteur" that is behind the drive for negative power. This Golden-Rule breaking, internal sabotaging outlaw is behind all aspects of the ongoing hubris that is hell bent on global suicide. Hindbrain culture is terminal as is now evidenced by the chickens of industrial civilization now all coming home to roost.

To achieve sovereignty we must gain distance from the negative-power pyramid so that the neurogenesis needed for higher executive functioning and Triune brain integration can occur. "Distance" or fair witnessing is achieved by going beyond the compartmentalization caused by our reactive interpretation of positive and negative. Attraction and aversion contract and tie up thought, emotion and behavior into habitual tracks that reduce both our perception of Reality and its spontaneous flow. We have defined our identity by our likes and dislikes, but have forgotten about the geni behind the curtain. If we step back from interpreting an emotion 'positive' or 'negative', the raw sensation of life - unfiltered, raw dynamic Presence energy floods our being. We then live from the Fair Witness, beyond the associative narrative of the story maker, to experience tacit measureless infinity. Then every thought, sensation, feeling, and impulse is infused with the mystery of the universe.

An amalgam of commodified parts—homogeny, fear, usury, sound bites and assimilated ideas—is not individualization. Compliance with, or rebellion from the Borg is not sovereignty. The cooked Borg is not in full possession of themselves due to numbness and dumbness, thus their drives, responses, ideas, feelings, sensory awareness and behaviors are conditioned and based on fictions of the future and dream-like memory of the past. Therefore if you fall into the low energy of the Borg's reality tunnel, you lose your Self and are degraded and shat on in some form or another. The sovereign works at creating openness, flexibility, clarity, purity, spontaneity, readiness and enthusiasm in mind and body in order to maintain "high-leverage opportunities" and a spiritualized trajectory.

If we fail to build up the neurophysiology of the inner Janus, then we cannot present our true Self in honesty, freedom and integrity to the world. If we are not being our true Self, then the socio-ecosystem or *milieu* we create around us is at odds with who we really are and where we want to go. The great danger of casual submission to the "Made" world, is that we are not actually living OUR life, but are actually existing in the default mode of gross existential compromise. We default on our sovereignty through allowing ourselves to be infected and infested by multitudinous alien realities. We must first recognize and know our Self before the universe can respond "appropriately" to our noble being and thereby uphold and preserve our integrity/integration. Our being must be permeated with exquisite self-empathy before we can love ourselves enough to consciously create our existence and experience from the inside out.

When we repress the frequencies of fear, anger, and grief arising from our past we remain unintegrated and this creates dissonance and dissociation in our flesh by which we are separated from our Presence and the present moment. Only in pure Presence are we capable of receiving the divinely luminous opportunity to intimately engage and explore our full HUman potential. Reacting to the power dynamics and machinations of the Borg will forever keep our neurology locked into a death grip with dysfunction. Ultimately it just feeds our powerlessness if we engage in trying to out wit, fight, control, get on top of or stop the negative power plays we encounter.

Complaining, self-righteousness and pointing the finger also do nothing to reinstate our sense of wellbeing and resolve toxic stress. Rather than attempting to find resolution, retribution or restitution the way to deal with the "unlove" of pathological power is to get out of the mind altogether and pull ones focus into the center…using practices such as the Heart-Tree Meditation. Liberation from the Borg involves disengaging from animal combat and leaving drama of human chaos behind through building and aligning with our integral core, by which we and the Universe are One. That is, in response to unlove the answer is always to "unify."

> *"No one is coming to save us from ourselves."* ~ Michael Brown

Michael Brown in his Presence Process says, only by consciously developing our capacity to "feel" are we delivered beyond the predicament of inauthenticity created by suppressing and sedating our unintegrated emotional condition. That is, we become whole by "feeling" rather than numbing the emotional intercommunication of the neocortex through the brain's spindle cell network. The spindle neuron cells are four times larger and very wide for carrying high velocity transmission. They are particularly thick between the orbitofrontal cortex (OFC) and the anterior cingulate cortex (ACC), from which the spindle cells extend to various parts of the brain, especially those areas associated with social behavior. Spindle neurons are rich in receptors for serotonin, dopamine and vasopressin—neurotransmitters involved in mood, bonding, love, fidelity, integrity, sincerity and pleasure.

The richly branched network of spindle cells orchestrate empathy in the OFC to elicit feelings, first impressions, flash decisions, recognition, likes and dislikes. The spindle cell superhighway governs social guidance, diplomacy, schmoozing, intimacy, social graces and social intelligence. Thus by frequently practicing the Heart-tree Meditation we pull ourselves out of the disrupting frequency of combat and return to the core Mother Tree by which we are made whole. When we are whole, no amount of monkey business coming our way can throw us off center…and it is from this still center that our sovereign Self-determinacy and true destiny grows

THE CLASH OF LEVELS

How to manage the disharmony of others around us during our awakening of kundalini, consciousness and sovereignty? As we "open" to greater sentience, we must simultaneously become stronger and more discerning of both inner and outer influences. All of us can only perceive phenomena from the meme level that we gravitate on, so it is pointless wasting our energy in righteous indignation as others try to drag our "goodness" through the mud. They cannot even see us, and what they don't understand they attack in order to try and control and profit. So in having a more expanded awareness we are continually having to extend goodwill and forgiveness to depraved and delinquent others who have no idea that they are actually operating in bad-will, because they are not sovereign informed.

Rather than being drawn down into the primitive fray by either responding to or trying to fix the unconscious, sub-sentient behavior of others—the sovereign must "use" the attack to become more fully alive and to quicken their own sovereign destiny. It is very easy to fall into a pit of social stress, self-pity, righteousness, martyrdom or even messianic retaliation in wanting to save people from their own fallen natures, but that is not respecting the "non-interference" principle of sovereignty law. *Each person must come to their own sovereign empowerment, under their own steam, in their own time.* So instead of being blown around in default by the Borg momentum, we must proactively and preemptively establish sovereign momentum that has break-away capacity from the reptilian power machinations on all levels — individual, groups, gender, state, and species

Since it is those of a higher level, the preceptors, geniuses and those that are already out of the conditioned matrix who have the broadest vision and the greatest potential for meta-skill building…it is up to us to process the ignorance, dysfunction, aggression, misunderstanding and outright nastiness of the revenge of the zombies. The higher we can establish our emotional equilibrium out of the shadow realm via illuminated prefrontal focus on the workings of our own reptilian (autonomic) functions, the less family, friends and coworkers will exercise their demons on us.

Due to the unending paranoia of those that are ignorant of the alchemy of awakening, we may not be able to work directly with them but instead must work upon our own understanding and energy, and seek Self satisfying expression with those on a similar wavelength. Substantiation of the sovereign brain does ironically take social reinforcement by peers who are naturally beneficent and live by The Golden Rule. The little egoic self feels trapped, vulnerable and exposed to the energies of awakening…and so we need to reassure those around us that "all is well" and give them enthusiastic encouragement as to their own unlimited potential.

It is not surprising that those entrenched in a thick cocoon tend to get belligerent, contrary, petty and self-serving around a fast transmuter. It is as though their shadow is coming out and the aggression they had towards their parents and the world, which was never allowed to be expressed, is now coming out and being directed at you. Of course to simply allow oneself to be put in martyr position is untenable. Radical exercise, dancing and outrageous humor with peers is necessary in order to release the tension presented by the impossibility of this and other kinds of social quicksand. Physical and emotional release is the first step in learning the social alchemical processes necessary to allow our own evolution in a presovereign, life-negating and anti-evolutionary society. If the shoe doesn't fit, don't wear it!

• THE CRIME OF SELF-NEGATION

Once we get that self-victimization is a crime against life by default, neglect and self-betrayal, then we are on the home stretch to the sovereign life. As a sovereign, we have a moral obligation to protect presovereigns' from destroying their souls by refusing to offer ourselves as a sacrificial lamb to their power addiction. The psychopath relies on the basic goodness of others in order to "feed." Thus by turning the polarities and refusing to be "good" in relation to the psychopath, then they can no longer feed and will run off in fear of their lives for their secret is blown.

Naming or calling the dragon out is the most up front, straightforward method, although often not applicable during workplace hierarchies. When there are restrictions that may threaten your immediate livelihood, then *questioning the dragon* is often a softer approach in dealing with psychopaths in the workplace. Questioning the dragon involves a slower method of gradually making it known that you are onto the wicked machinations of the psychopath and that you will not simply capitulate to being eaten alive.

Self-negation is a form of spiritual suicide, due to the "self" effectively ceasing to exist as a proactive agent. The use of negative power is only dropped when sovereignty of the individual is the fundamental social and socializing principle, for only then are we truly HUman. Having grown up in self-defeating, poverty-minded homes, the presovereign adult may be inclined to undervalue play by being too focused on scarcity and limitation. Allegiance to false doctrines that are not in alignment with our highest ideals and desires, can only lock us into a life of self-negation and self-betrayal.

"Tyranny, in this model, is not created by tyrants alone but by neurotic masses who want tyrants." ~ Wilhelm Reich

SOCIAL INNER ART PRACTICES
The following exercises will help to not only substantiate our own core Self, but will also help us transmute any social dis-ease we may encounter.

•RELEASING/FORGIVING
Letting go of the victim's attachment to hurt and blame Aka cords with others is an organic process of cellular forgiveness which may be necessary to include in a daily practice until it is not an issue anymore. This releasing of others is vitally important in order to free up one's energy to activate the cerebral cortex and initiate heart-brain integration. Realizing our sovereignty is one and the same as letting go of over sensitivity, victimhood, helplessness, enmeshment, and codependency. Lie on your back with your head turned to the left. Get into the receptive (change) state by dropping the back of the tongue, doing the Inner Smile and belly breathing.

With your right hand press into the ascending colon on the right side of your lower belly. With the left hand cup your fingers under the left ribcage and press into the spleen. Focus on an emotional trigger with another individual and feel the body letting go, forgiving and forgetting the issue. Set the other free in love and compassion, refusing to burden them any longer with your angst. To release someone you have previously been attached to from your energy field, send him or her energetically away like seeing off a friend on a ship, while you are standing in a stream or the ocean. Listen to Michael Beckwith's Revisioning CD #2 on Victimhood.

• RELEASING WALK
Go for a barefoot walk nature and cock your head to the left, as you breathe out, do so with a huff through the nose. Periodically take three deeper breaths and huff out forcefully through the mouth. While you do this forcefully flap your hands as though you are shaking water off of them. Each time your mind wants to go over hurt, blame, justice and self-righteous tapes cock your head the left and huff it out of you. Know that when you cellularly forgive someone they start behaving more human. But you cannot truly forgive someone with your mind, so it is pointless ruminating. By stopping stressful recycling of social conflict in your head and huffing the tension out of your body you give the relationship room to evolve. You can use social conflict as grit to create the pearl of your sovereignty. It is the unskillful means of not claiming our full humanity that causes delinquent, dysfunctional and delusional behavior.

When we resonate in sovereignty in the presence of the "disempowered" they may start to become sane. Releasing conflict through the cellular transcendence of tension allows us to become increasingly whole in a world of escalating chaos. The divide between the immorality and injustice of conventional culture, and the transpersonal morality of the awakened is going to become increasingly obvious….and so we must use this polarity to our advantage. When we observe a lack of humanity and ethics, we can use our Heart as a compass pointing directly to Universal Law and increased humaneness. We can thus grow our Fair Witness, remove our triggers and increase the Light by transmuting the darkness rather than resonating with it, running from it or fighting it.

"Small minds can't comprehend big spirits. To be great, you have to be willing to be mocked, hated, and misunderstood. Stay strong."
~ Robert Tew

• ATTRACTION MEDITATION

This practice is for changing polarity from self-abandonment, self-rejection, and repulsion, to fulfillment and receptivity. When we fill up from source by turning the polarity of our love inward, we become satiated and our world is reenchanted. Sit spine erect in meditation and take off the top of your head by making a plane through your head at the eyebrow level. This puts your inner kinesthetic senses at this plane…then let the energy of Universe pour into your head along your body's magnetic flux lines. This produces greater connection of one's EMF-egg and the coherent organization and alignment of all bodies and levels up to the Unified Field.

Usually when we meditate we are projecting our energy up and out, but when we flip the polarity and let Universe pour inwards, the kundalini gland at the base of the spine starts pulsing (you can feel this if you are lying on your back in bed during this exercise). This inner spark represents greater connection between the top and bottom of our EMF-egg. You can also open up your head to the lines of force pouring in from Universe while you are doing upright walking. This gives a strange fixity and intensity to the vision and makes monkey mind disappear in pure awareness.

Pure awareness is quantum consciousness, while normal awareness is digital. You will notice that is maximally energetic and you will have to breathe deeper in order to maintain the groove of open headedness while doing upright walking. Rising up to your correct stature in life includes straightening your spine so that your brain can be fed with the full force of your glorious energy. The "trance" produced from Upright Walking in combination with the Attraction Meditation and feeling the EMF egg enter the crown — is not so much a trance but the absence of trance. That is our normal daily mind and personality is actually a trance state, while upright walking in the noble posture with the eyes at the horizon or above allows the brain to be fully fed which drops the monkey-mind ego, so that pure unadulterated awareness is perceived.

Consciously working with the Law of Attraction is the first baby step towards proactively living the Muse to manifest a life in tune with our highest values and greatest joy. When we focus on techniques, material possessions or success by power-over methods we can never be secure. Only in living true to the highest within us can we ever hope to feel at home in our body and realize a deeper relationship with nature.

• SERPENT KISSING LOVERS

This meditation is the first of the advanced sovereignty building exercises. Lie on your back in bed or on the ground in nature. Place the right hand under the left breast with the thumb point up on the sternum; place the left hand cupping the right ribcage over the liver with the thumb pointing up on the sternum. Now feel-sense a caduceus inside the body with the double helix going up the spine and the two snake heads as the brain hemispheres. Focus attention on the top of the forehead and sense a kissing of the hemispheres at the crest of the forehead. This is done in association with active dropping of discursive thought and inner/outer conflicts by focusing peace into the brainstem, opening the heart to the forebrain and breathing into areas in the body that are blocked or numb.

As the charge builds up there is a very real sense of maturity, parenting, royalty, rulership, empowerment and one pointed attention. You will need to breath deeply to assimilate and contain the intense power generated. If it is dark you might see two merging light balls with the inner eye, which ultimately form into one ball of light. The Kissing Lovers sexercise essentially allows a nondual alchemical means of overcoming ego and conditioning and to transcend stress and disorder by working through all that stands in the way of this sublime integration. Crossing the hands over on opposite sides of the body acts to further ground the charge, as in the Egyptian death pose!

The Inner Arts work to elevate the nervous system beyond pathological power programming. It is hard to do this by oneself, as the human is a social animal. Spiritual gains are most often a solo affair, but spiritual maintenance and substantiation occurs largely through the mirrored reflection of like minds, in a face-to-face interaction—thus we must learn new patterns of relating that reinforce the sovereign state of ourselves and others.

• VIRTUAL REUNION

To help soften the heart and eliminate subliminal sadness and closure we can feel-imagine meeting the significant others in our life. This is great done in the bath, in bed or a special place in nature where you can be alone. Start off with the person you love the most and imagine the time and place you would meet this particular person and give them a virtual hug. Allow your heart to experience the full cascade of emotion, don't cut it short and move onto the next person until you feel a sense of resolution and balance.

You can do this with deceased relatives, family, friends, enemies or anyone you feel a sense of separation and non-completion with. It could take you days or years to process just one person so don't hurry. The fact that you are seeking reunion and the rejoining of love is what matters. The whole world will feel your virtual reunion practice…of unconditional love and acceptance and return to the heart. What you focus on grows, so CHOOSE the highest for you, and don't look at the cracks in the pavement. Commit to creating higher energy levels for yourself by dancing in the new world.

• KING AND QUEEN POSE

Lie in the Egyptian death pose with arms crossed over chest and meditate directing ones eyeballs and mind's eye into the brainstem. Since it is Betawave consciousness that usurps our energy and creates dissonance in the autonomic nervous system, putting our energy and attention into the brain stem calms this area down, allowing a systems coherence needed to draw on higher levels of consciousness, thereby increasing steadiness, centeredness and nobility. Brainstem meditation is good for centering, soul recovery, boundary formation and general healing and wholing. Perhaps it focuses consciousness in the occipital lobes which are serotonin based, contributing to integration and harmony. The King and Queen state of our innate nobility, is the source of our confidence, swagger and agency.

• THE ROYAL HELM

Along with the King and Queen Pose this practice will help to grow you into your center and generate the cohesion necessary for self-dominion. While lying on your back (in bed) press the thumbs together facing upwards over the sternum with the hands crossed over and cupped like the wings of a dove over the ribs under the breasts. This provides loving, warm emotional support to the diaphragm muscle. Now focus the mind's eye at the top of the forehead to establish the royal Uraeus. While drawing energy to the point at the top of the forehead silently repeat such phrases as: "I am the executor, I am the decider, I am the ruler of my life." Even the Emerald Tablet is code for inner arts meditation.

• POSITIVE PROJECTION PRACTICE (PPP)

This involves greater intimacy with our psychic and spiritual levels by incorporating Inner Arts, meditation, breathing, dreams, active imagination and good-will. By doing PPP regularly you are setting the energetic template for change and evolution to occur. Then evolvement will spontaneously occur in the "space" you have cleared with your Pollyanna imagination. In bed prior to sleep is a good time to focus on this and taking melatonin prior to PPP amplifies the experience and benefits. Build the connection between the opening heart and the prefrontal lobes using slow deep breathing, with one hand on the heart the other on the solar plexus.

Keep the mind's eye focused on the prefrontal lobes and draw energy up the back of your head. Take any conflict that is pressing on you and see the Other and yourself operating from the sovereign perspective. Don't bother trying to find solutions right now, just focus on building the "energy" of transcendence related to the sovereign solution. While generating the Heart-PFL plasma connection you can do the Inner Smile, Inner Candle or the V For Humor practice.

Positive play, that is not mere escapism, is the elixir of youth and the greatest source of inspiration for productivity and happiness.

• SUBSTANTIATING THE HOLOGRAPHIC SELF

Rather than shunning the earthy, ignorant and less evolved levels of humanity, we can "use" them perversely for our own evolution. Meaning that, in working through that which triggers us into a "contractive" response we can become more transparent to the light. The less we hold onto, the more light is conveyed through every crevice of our being. If we do not actually exercise our ability to remain transparent to light and a pure vehicle for our soul, we have no idea how deep down the rabbit hole of the universe we go.

• BUILDING LEFT-BRAIN EFFICACY

For improved/increased critical thinking skills build up the left brain do ambidextrous and binaural exercises like juggling, dancing and moving barefoot over rocky ground, balance bar etc... Chess, brain-teasers, backgammon, planning, writing, math, logic puzzles, complex computer programs, scrabble, and even spelling drills — any sorts of exercises that prioritize the factual, concrete and associative, as well as personal narrative are among the best left brain exercises. Study of the classical curriculum—Trivium: grammar, logic, and rhetoric. Quadrivium: comprising of the four liberal arts of number, geometry, music, and cosmology. For left-brain ordering read Ken Wilber. For increasing efficiency in your daily life read Tim Ferris.

• SIMS OF SOCIAL SUCCESS

Visualize the way you want to be and the way you want others to treat you. Make these simulations as lively and emotionally vivid as possible; incorporating sensation and enthusiastic exaggerated body movements. Through visual simulations we can proactively and positively impact our social experience and break through patterns of hesitance, shyness, conflict, defense, paradoxical intention, confusion and duplicit will. Simulation practice helps get all our parts and levels lined up and moving in the same direction. The brain registers the visualization (simulations) as real as far as brain activity goes...this means we can experience success through inner practice, which makes it more likely that social fluidity and connection will occur in the real world.

Our reality is as plastic as our determination and skill at changing it. Felt simulations of success allow us to become masters of our own will...which makes it more likely that others will have confidence in us and feel connected. Simulations of success is one of the best ways of living the future now, through faithfulness (high fidelity) to the unique Self. Differentiation from the "collective" insures our thrival, and not just mere survival. Without bringing online our visionary capacities we have little control over the reactionary, automatic, default nature of the cause and effect world and our own will.

The science and art of redemption requires the understanding of emotions and their compassionate elevation, regulation and cultivation.

• PLEASURE OF DEVILRY

Unless you can give the Borg immediate satisfaction in the form of money, status, position, sex, security, entertainment, food and addictive substances the Hindbrain human will try and extract pleasure via underhanded, aggressive and wicked means. Humor ~ positive humor that is, being a prefrontal lobe function that tantalizes the Hindbrain, cuts through the evil delight and negative intent of Borg machinations. Humor is one of the few options available to dealing with the Borg in a positive, proactive manner, without being devolved by the twisted nature of the lower mind.

Unless you can nip devilry in the bud with humor the compulsive Borg invariably has to escalate with evil projections, unfair judgments, false accusations, group bullying, stories, lies, tricks and other various means of attack and subterfuge. The stronger their attack the more they have to justify their behavior and the less likely they are to admit to they are sociopathic.

• DEALING WITH SUBVERSIVE HUMOR

Monkeys love to throw shit at each other. The general default mode of behavior in a stressed prepersonal society is to try and get one over on others through subversive humor. To deal with this common problem we can take the stance of pre-emptive social cleansing—to purify the bathwater for the poor fellows through magnanimous humor. One of the greatest challenges for the sovereign is to first not take such insults personally, or be put out and disheartened… and then to give the gift of love by boosting the attackers self-esteem without diminishing ourselves, or acting in self-righteous one-upmanship. That is we return the bad-will joke with a good-will joke without sarcasm, flattery or defense. Enlivening social engagement raises the bar.

• TURNING SHIT INTO ROSES

We move forward despite negative emotion. Half of life may be a bed of roses, but the roses are growing in composted shit. If we don't tend the soil, the roses will not bloom so well. Social aikido can be called "Turning Shit into Roses." We cannot get very far with our development in sovereignty until we master this transmuting social alchemy. For the prefrontal lobes will not open and stabilize if we are being pulled down into nerve shattering reflexes to daily insults. I found out about this "play angle" when I accidentally didn't register the nasty dig that someone gave me, and I came back immediately with a huge magnanimous response.

This cut the predator/prey dynamic short and the aggressor didn't get his demonic glee, but was raised to befuddled heights by my sparkling comeback. Practice turning shit into roses with your friends first, so that you can build up your capacity to stay in the Good Parent mode while under fire. Remember the subversive predator will always try and catch you off-guard and so you must build your artful response as the automatic default reflex mode of the new sovereign you.

When you move towards an experience, it comes and it goes. When you avoid or back away from an experience it can hang around forever. Another way of saying that is what you resist persists. The mind is often an instrument of resistance as we try to avoid certain difficult sensations in our body. The more mindfully we orient ourselves to the world, the less the mind, (and reactivity stored in the mind) dominates and disorients the being. When you avoid an experience it can hang around forever, repeating again and again. Completing what has been incomplete in your life clears the way for the new and the unusual to occur, as we raise our energy valence higher and higher. *Post Borgism = Compost that shit! Sovereignty = Own your shit!*

• REMAINING CONSCIOUS

This is perhaps one of the most important skills for the emerging sovereign to develop, because we are dealing with that split second in which the anaesthetizing and stress chemicals flood the brain and illicit either a knee jerk reaction in kind or a passive systems shutdown. If we can remain conscious through breath, circulating the energy charge, and taking the tension off of the heart then we can instantly come from the place of dominion and elicit the most beneficent response, unique to each situation. Enlivening, and fortifying our felt-presence in our forehead establishes a potently alive commanding Uraeus. As we deepen and mature our sovereignty practice we become more centered in the kinesthetic interoceptive sense of the prefrontal cortex and emerge triumphant through the awesome connecting power of presence.

Turning shit into roses helps others realize that they too do not have to shit in their own bathwater and to suffer the cruel sense of separation that results from their bellicose displays of false power and belligerence. They know not what they do, but we can lead the way by turning our our headlights. The Tao te Ching says there is no greater misfortune than underestimating your enemy by dismissing him as evil. For thereby you destroy your three treasures "compassion," "frugality," and "humility," and become an enemy yourself.

• STANCE OF SOCIAL IMMUNITY

The way to approach disharmonious harmful vibrations is to fully acknowledge them, but to learn not resonate in their frequency. To do this you need a transpersonal, transanthropic "scientific" viewpoint and to maintain universal objectivity throughout all the days of your life. It is rather hard to be reactive and get pulled into and bound up in Mara (illusion/evil/desire/aversion) when you see and feel everything from a Universal vibration. Rather than the simplistic notion of non-judgment, you clearly see the "devilish" mechanism of the evil intent (bite/trigger/dig), but you do not get sucked in to believing that it has any relevance to you and where you are going.

You can rationally work out what is happening, by looking at human affairs through primate psychology dynamics and learning the neurochemistry involved. Plainly stating what people are doing to their face, is likely to just cause more trouble than it is worth, by engaging the negative ego of the other still further. But by knowing the neurochemistry of human primate dynamics we can use skillful means to recover our own connection, strength and center. With mindful distance we can then utilize such tools as energy, consciousness, camouflage (clothing), the power of the voice, breath, exercise, nature, sunlight and Presence in a non-reactive, non-confrontational fashion. This way you can distance yourself from the present machinations of Borg affairs in order to "cut through it" like a knife, rather than getting caught up in the mess.

With mastery a temporary dissonant note in the almighty hum of the Universal song soon turns with the Tao back to resonance. As we deal with the collective shadow in an alchemical fashion, this allows the ongoing creation of new internal technologies to deal with madness, stress, shadow and repression, thereby permitting evolution, maturity and stabilization of the sovereign Self. Pain is there to tell you what to do, if you awaken to its message.

• CONFRONTATION AND DISCLOSURE

The growth towards sovereignty requires a direct accountability and inquiry of the perpetrator by the victim, or both sides remain polarized in the sadomasochistic trance, and continue to infect their future with the power-disease of the past. Directly facing off with a power-abuser is essential to moving on, rather than relying on endless displacement activity...talks with therapists, numbing addictions, endless hurt/blame mental rumination, revenge or appealing to higher authority. You may have to first get some distance from the wounding situation to muster the equanimity, reserves and resolve to confront someone who may have tortured you for years. But you cannot grow in mental, physical and spiritual strength and resolve toxic stress unless you bring the clandestine social pathology out into the light of day and have your say.

• GELASSENHEIT

Grokking and open relating or the practice of Gelassenheit, (*letting-go and letting-be*), is a compassionate style of listening meditation and social interaction that comes more from "allowing" the Heart/Right-Brain wiring to gain prominence; rather than dissecting analysis of our interpersonal interactions through the left-brain's narrative and status preoccupations. We thus enter "We Space" through the empathetic circuitry by first training ourselves to love our own flesh and our own core by turning the Mind's Eye within to deeply feel our innate a priori health, thereby restoring the connection between feeling, listening and allowing. Growing up in presovereign, dependent families we were taught to look for love and attention outside of ourselves, and so we remain starved of our own affection, health and integration our entire lives. Once we have unconditionally reconnected with ourselves and established the hardware for Grokking, we can then drop the safety-judgment monitoring system (vigilance) of the left-brain's security narrative.

Energy and consciousness that was formerly spent in "scanning for safety and status" can then be channeled into feeling, openness and allowing. The energy that was spent in the paranoia of power differential can then be spent in Grokking, hearkening, or the fully embodied flow of holistic perception... similar to **Gendlin's focusing or Zen's shikantaza.** This felt-sense mode of perception permits the mystic connection within and without by restoring the bodily felt-sense of deep listening without the inertia of repression, resistance or rejection. In other words, we need to cultivate a listening that is deeply rooted in our body's felt sense of being situated fully in the present, with spacious knowing, patience and tolerance for silence and the unknown. Thus permitting the coherent synchronization and reception of information by all the various modes of sensory antennae. By relating within and without through the opened empathetic circuitry we can then reintegrate those parts of us that have been cut off and deadened, thus recovering our full resources, full senses, full health and deep humanity.

• COMPASSIONATE PRAYER

Prayerful meditation focused on the health and well-being of an individual or all sentient beings, is a principle method of developing the middle prefrontal lobes. As we meditate on say, the enhancement of another person's immune system, a warm ball of light is felt at the third eye and the solar plexus. As we prime ourselves for compassionate action on another's behalf, Gamma waves are generated in the middle of the prefrontal lobes. This undoubtedly is the maximum frequency for sending "God Force" instantaneously through the aether to establish a healing connection. If you do this don't tell the person you are doing it for unless you know for sure they would be receptive.

Compassionate meditation for others is also the highest frequency for the spontaneous healing of our own mind, heart and health. It is especially effective when directed at people we are out of sorts with or those on the opposite side of the fence. Prayerful meditation is so effective because it reestablishes our alignment with the Unitive Force...for in essence there is no separation once we re-member it is so. In this way rejection of the Self is undone. In Vedic times Brahman meant the power inherent in prayer, later in the Upanishad era it came to be known as the cosmic reality underlying the phenomenal world.

• RIGHT LIVELIHOOD

When you sell evolutionary product(s) that humanity needs to get through this "eye of the needle," then you no longer need to make a living through the normal channels of healing, spirituality, teaching, information dispersal etc... This frees up our service to others (dharma) from the corruption and inertia associated with acquiring money exchange. This is the fastest route to the new socio-economy and post-formal ethics. It is also the fastest route to establishing the financial liquidity needed to grow and develop ourselves so that our spiritual vocation is actualized and successful. Things are changing rapidly now, we need to figure out where we fit in and jump into the fast moving stream. We shouldn't fear the pace of change, for this speed is releasing us from a past which is no longer working for us. The sooner we let go of the immaturity and moral bankruptcy of the Borg, the faster the new way comes into being. Certainty on doing the "right thing" and remaining true to the Muse will carry us through, when we seek direction from the silence within..

• TRULY SERVING OTHERS

With those still embedded in the Matrix we cannot "save" them from the collapsing civilization or their own physical, mental emotional developmental corruption. We are ALL refugees in transition from the death culture to the living culture. Rapid habit change away from our addiction to the death culture is what is needed, and we each have to come back to "Life" of our own choosing. There is a lot of pain, numbness and self-betrayal to move through for most people and they have to relearn how to relate to themselves, others and the earth in a power-equity way. In the death culture we keep our suffering and denial under a thick layer of sadomasochism, ie: the infliction or reception of pain or humiliation. The adrenaline and endorphin "hit" we get from power-abuse and being abused acts like a drug that produces a loss of feeling, disconnection and a loss of sentience. This "power anesthetic" brings about a reversible loss of consciousness…but the more "hits" of power abuse we experience in our daily life, or the more negative attachment we are to extracting status stress from others…the less likely we are to evolve out of the Hindbrain state and save ourselves from going down with the death culture.

• THE GIFT OF GRACE

Initiation, transmutation, transformation takes a lifetime and is an alchemical continuum across the generations of time. The greatest "gift" we have to offer others is the depth of our own Presence. We cannot walk other people's path for them. And we cannot teach anyone anything, as long as we haven't reached it ourselves and achieved gnosis on our own. Commercial spirituality is little more than intellectual knowledge passed from one person to another. There is no point in it; in fact, it causes more harm than good—empty endless circles that waste our time, strength, hopes, money and energy and only to lead us further away from ourselves and our direct connection with our spirit. Spiritual connection (gnosis, Jhana) always descends upon us from above, directly into our being through our own readiness to open. We can however be an enthusiastic catalyst for grace in others through our surrender to apotheosis, for spirit is contagious. All good, truth and beauty arises from a prior existing effortless grace-of-being afforded by Original Blessing.

Enthusiasm is the ensouling of your heart-mind with your passion, self-integrity, "heart-felt" values, universal principles, visions and inspired action. (*Enthusiasm* = en (*within*) + theos (*god*) = "having the god within.")

• SELF-HATRED, THE PRINCIPLE POISON

In our misemployed and cheapened state as an industrial prostitute, no matter how hard we try we can never give enough to satisfy the insane hunger of a spiritually deficient society. We are taught to hate ourselves because we can only offer an insignificant insufficient, contribution when we are not actively engaged in the unique genius of our soul vocation. Thus both we and our community remain unsatisfied and unfulfilled, and stuff the gapping hole with collective substance abuse, complaining and backbiting. By crawling on top of each other we substitute power-abuse for empowerment.

This invalidation and spiritual misalignment is why self-hatred is systemic within commercially driven cultures. So transfixed are we by the the paycheck from the company and the thankless job that we fail to ask what we really want from life. How can we get what we want or achieve our dreams if we are not 100% clear on what they are?

The stress of the lie we lead keeps us in the slave state, void of the passion, vitality and motivation to break free from the chain gang. When we fail to engage the circuitry for sovereignty and self-dominion we participate in, indeed we initiate our own downfall and obsolescence. By embracing the ultimate limitation of self-hatred we stop the entropic waste of lifeforce spent in trying to fit into a life we don't even want and discover the endless reserves of love by which we can create a life beyond anything we could have hoped for in our broken quasi-voluntary slavery.

• ENCOURAGING OTHERS TO FIND THEIR OWN WAY

Karmically it is up to each individual to find their own way home to their sovereign or divine self. Your ship will sink if you disrespect the sovereignty of others and try to be Source for them, rather than encouraging them to find their own sustenance from Source. Thus it is more important to encourage others to find themselves, than to offer them advise, solutions or directions. We can however offer travel hints, especially those of a fundamental nature such as detoxification and raw-regeneration.

Thus getting friends, family and colleagues to watch Youtube videos by David Wolfe, Dan McDonald, Dr Robert Morse, Brian Clement and Gabriel Cousens, M.D. may be a way to "truly serve others" without encroaching on their sovereign rights to be delinquent and degenerating if they so desire. **Inspiratio per Exemplum.** or *"Inspiration through Example"* is the way into the beneficent future without upsetting or demoralizing the apple cart and generating resistance to truth of the Life Force. Emphasis should always be on our own right attitude, right thought, right action, right livelihood etc... Because at the end of the day we cannot fix, nor help anyone but ourselves, and on doing so we change the world.

"To find your own way is to follow your bliss." ~ Joseph Campbell

SELF-CARE FOR SOCIAL STRESS

"Love connects with love. But love should never subvert itself to a lower standard in order to accommodate another person's dysfunction." ~ Gary Null

Just as physical immunity is important to the preservation of the self, so too is social immunity, and so we have to create a lifestyle that fosters conditions in which we can BE ourselves. If we are not being and expressing who we really are, we will always be vulnerable to maligned forces, for we ourselves are misaligned. If we are our Self, we are resilient no matter what kind of shadow projection comes our way. For at least we have the authentic joy of the cosmic connection of the Self if we stand strong against the caustic degradating nature of Hindbrain social antics. We have little capacity to change other people, especially when they are operating out of the Hindbrain. However don't let the retardation of presovereign Hindbrains affect and infect your light.

Engage in meditative, healing and exercise practices in nature on the grass, rocks, beach or water. The body is trying to normalize, or rather optimize itself, and cannot do so without nature's energies. If you are not using Nature's energies forget trying to optimize or normalize cause it an't going to happen. Modern man has everything stacked against him — cooked food, EMFs, media poisoning, corrupt system, GMOs, radiation etc...

We are hit by discombobulating "noise" on every front…while only Nature has the frequencies to harmonize and make us feel grounded, sane and well. So we need to consider using nature, the elements, breathing, living-water and earthing as FOOD, in order to fill our body up electromagnetically more-so than with food itself. Food to the body suffering from negation and deficit disorder just makes us feel more hungry and exhausted, because it is actually Nature's vital energies that our body is after. Principally…lying on the grass to earth the body whenever you feel weird helps to rebalance enough to reorient you on the Phi path.

We avoid doing the work of sovereign realization when stuck in "victim, angel, martyr, messiah" mode, because we are in "reactivity" to social-persecution and usury. If we are putting energy into self-reinforcement, self-defense and self-justification, this is stemming from our survival circuits and so we get locked into a polar reactive response to the Borg, internally fighting external shadow. When we are in flight or fight we are not in Wholebrain mode and so we cannot establish sovereign integration (integrity)…this confounds the synergy needed for the Soul-ution.

Disenfranchisement provides the opportunity to find our strength within a dark, disempowering system. Once conditioned into submission and powerlessness the broken individual has no way of breaking out of the cage that was created for us. The disempowered individual embedded in the sadomasochistic trance cannot detoxify their nervous system, clear their mind and draw on inner resources to express their whole, integrated and purposeful being. The way through blockage, resistance and opposition is to raise your energy level and presence till the miasma becomes softened, transparent and can be released. As a sovereign our emotional freedom resides in knowing that we cannot change another, but we can change ourselves. When the stickiness of other people's reality puts us in retreat and stagnation, we have to push through social glue to generate lively productive movement. Cooperation means ascent on the atomic, cellular, organ and interpersonal level. We go to God together or not at all.

Sacrifice, denial, negation and silencing of our truth as opposed to the actualization of the Self lies at the core of the cultural consensus of spiritual retardation. Spiritual denial is the default condition of Borg culture. And it takes a deliberate effort to break through the denial and take a breath of fresh air, to really see what is really going on. To be sovereign is to be nonviolent and non-violating having transcended the sadomasochistic use of consciousness… preserving our own nobility and the dignity of others who would sin against us. Allowing a bully, parasite or predator to continually feed on us without addressing and stopping the situation is cowardice, it is not strength.

"Without sufficient self-defense, peace is nothing but an unattainable dream. Similarly, lovers cannot love others unless they feel secure enough to love themselves first. If your life is full of the devastating emotions of anger and defeat because you have left yourself wide open for the taking, then it will be very difficult to have positive emotions towards others. You will begin to resent all people, because in your eyes they are vicious, and they are all thieves." Thick Face, Black Heart, Chin-Ning Chu.

Getting beyond the sound barrier of compliance to presovereign social dynamics means we must remove the blocks to our enthusiasm and eliminate the lies, automatic habits and knee-jerk reactions to The Given concourse of human interactions. When we first begin to actively change our conditions in support of the development of the sovereign brain, we may need to undertake a regime of physical exertion, nootropic supplements and psychoactive herbs to increase the honesty of our Truth Speak. This is so because our patterns of self-suppression will continue to create Hindbrain social circumstances that necessitate unauthenticity and lying to others and ourselves.

A lack of honesty and forthrightness in our speech and behavior will prevent us from creating a social environment that supports the sovereignty of all individuals. If we fail to stand our sovereign ground and stoop to meet people at their level—their level may be so retarded and immoral that we get dragged into the muck. So rather than stooping we should stand tall and draw people up towards the light through the shocking power of truth, without appeasement, or the pitiful need for acceptance and without the ball breaking need to always be NICE!

Rather than getting angry at people's infantilism, codependency and sociopathy we can learn ways of behaving and communicating from our noble center that encourages others to act from their empowered noble center also. The key point is that when people are projecting darkness onto us, we must turn it around to generate more light. In this way the negative energy of other people's Hindbrain becomes our advanced positive Forebrain.

Those that hold latent psycho-spiritual power are subconsciously terrorized into a straight-jacket of self-suppression by the arrogance and caustic nature of sadomasochistic power-over and usury. Ignorance of the toxicity of negative power status differential is still almost 100% and so it goes on unabated for millennia. The repressed multitude hold their atomic power back and make themselves small to fit into the existing prison planet. It is up to us to set ourselves free. *To be free of using, is to be free.*

Social immunity incorporates, psychological, behavioral, physiological and organizational adaptations. Sovereigns have an optimistic attribute bias towards seeing the positive repercussions and opportunities in events as they have a self-acquired license for infinite growth. To maintain a strong resourced, enthusiastic, energetic advantaged position requires on-going training. Strenuous exercise especially of a martial kind and spontaneous physical expression like dance, as well as singing and toning act like a truth serum to disinhibit vocal expression largely by loosening armor, removing stagnation, raising metabolism and increasing oxygen. Light a candle, put on some soft mystical music and take a long bath with Epsom salts. Do this at least every second day for a while. Drink extra water when processing social stress up to 5 qts a day.

Hang over a bar 5 minutes a day, lie on the grass 1/2 hour a day doing breathing, take long walks in nature if possible. Social tension (especially shock) tends to get caught in the glut muscles, so bend your knees – stick your ass out and wiggle it like a duck. It is the running impulse that is being fired up, so the best thing would be to actually go for a run. Rolling on tennis balls on the floor also works for the gluts, plus spinal rolling with a **Fabrication Enterprises Cando Inflatable Roller** 7" x 17" and a Aerial Yoga Swing. While slightly bent jump from foot to foot real fast as though you were warming up for a game of sports. Daily stretching preferably on the grass, foot stomping, door frame pushing and boxing motions coordinating the whole body.

Check out the **Maori Haka war chant** videos on the web. Beat on your chest like a gorilla while making gorilla sounds. Focus on rooting your energy into the ground through your feet, build the sense of a cord going through you and extending out the top your head to infinity, and generate energy in your Hara. Also to work the tension out the gluts lie on your back and push your legs against a wall or tree. Eat extra greens and sprouts. Take 1/4 tsp of magnesium citrate with a large glass of water prior to bed if you are constipated, which often happens when we are under some form of persecution. Do drumming and go dancing, find someone to laugh with, check out new environs, a new movie, and get some positive stimulation, intellectual adventure and discovery.

> "No matter how convenient it seems, don't blindly submit to a bully's aggression. It may seem like the path of least resistance, but when you yield to his attacks, you encourage repeat bullying. Don't reward him for attacking you." kickbully.com

NUTRASYNTHETIC RADICAL HONESTY:

Nutraceutical substances that increase truthful expression are Iodine, Kelp, Oxytocin, Testosterone, DMAE, DHEA, Piracetam, Huperzine, Vinpocetine, Arginine, Acetyl L-Carnitine and L-Lysine, Dimethylglycine, N-Acetyl-Cysteine, Niacin, Ribose, and Phosphatidylserine.

AGENCY WILL POWER HERBS

TRUTH TELLING HERBS:

Rosemary, Thyme, Gotu Kola, Cedar, Coca leaves, Tribulus, Mucuna pruriens, Tongkat Ali, Bala, Nutmeg, Hungarian Parsley seed, Tulsi Basil, Chamomile, Cinnamon, Cardamom, Sassafras, Syrian rue, Solomon Seal Root, Peach leaves, Lemongrass, Deer's Tongue, Olive leaf, Japanese knotweed, Ginkgo.

One or two capsules of Mucuna pruriens, Banisteriopsis caapi, Tongkat Ali and Ginkgo powder can be taken prior to a need to assert boundaries or truth telling. Use this dopamine enhancing mix as a herbal social laxative in order to substantiate the new level of emancipation. Obviously the shamanic use of entheogens like Ayahuasca, Iboga and Psilocybin in a ceremonial or natural setting would serve to liberate us from toxic social patterns and past trauma. However, here I am suggesting that supplements and herbs be used on daily basis to raise personal empowerment, emotional strength, will and honest self-expression. Remineralization, enzymes, greens, raw-plant protoplasm, probiotics, aphrodisiacs, and herbs and supplements that increase cognition will all increase our enthusiasm, capacity for change, spontaneity, and the expression of our authentic Sovereign Self.

Sex hormone herbs and supplements, along with dopamine enhancing supplementation forms the basis of the **sovereignity pharmaneutrocopeia**. Sex hormone potency IS life potency and the agency and power to effect change in accord with the dictates of Eros. Keeping our sex hormones pumped up to youthful levels with herbs, supplements and practices is even more important for those who are celibate and not in a relationship. Without the potentization of a sexual relationship we have to try harder through exercise, spiritual practices and nutrition to maintain the hormonal base to our unique creativity, personal will and sovereignty. Nature dictates that *sex hormone potency* reflects the viability, functionality, sustainability, efficaciousness, power, strength, sufficiency, use, vigor and virtue of an organism.

POWER HERBS For Smoothies-Capsules- Tinctures:

Cacao, Catuaba bark, Clavo Huasca, Yohimbe, Suma Root, Maca, Mucuna, Mesquite, Muira Puama, Goji berries, Rhodiola, Aswagandha, Astragalus, Tongkat ali, Forskolin, Fo-Ti, Shilajit, Tribulus, Bacopa, Galangal, Shatavari, Sarsaparilla, Saw palmetto. Gotu Kola, Gingko, Garcinia cambogia, Celastrus seed, Kratom, Rehmannia root, Cistanche, Schisandra, Cnidium seed, Dodder seed, Horny Goats Weed, Nettle leaf, Asian ginseng (Panax ginseng), Siberian ginseng (Eleutherococcus), Chaga, Lion's Mane, Reishi, Maitake, Citrus aurantium, Coptis Root, Echinacea, Bilberry, Alfalfa, Oat or Barley grass, Mulberry leaf, Moringa, Kelp, Irish moss, Spirulina. Mutamba, Cat's Claw, Devil's Claw and Myrrh gum powder helps reduce the candida, insulin resistance, prediabetic foundations of Metabolic X that undermines sexual and creative potency

CHAPTER 12

WAKING UP AND SHOWING UP

Given the right circumstances, understanding and nutrition periods of fog and cognitive incapacitation during acute kundalini cycles can ultimately resolve and lead to general increased physical, subtle, psychic and causal capacities. Since we live in a mineral and phytochemically depleted civilization and have pro-inflammatory bodies, kundalini awakening can lead to permanent brain and organ damage if steps are not taken to detoxify, protect and strengthen. The neurogenesis stimulated by the extreme love-chemistry of awakening and the heightening of hormones, neurotransmitters and nerve activity permits us a taste of higher human functioning and greater capacities of consciousness, sensing, feeling and knowing that are undreamed of in so-called "normal" society. As we learn to create bodies specially conducive to awakening and utilizing our innate full HUman capacities, we will have less catastrophic spiritual crises with little metabolic fallout and damage.

If we are not allowed to think for ourselves how are we to learn? How can we be awake to Reality if our bodyminds are built for non-sentience, non-sense, nonsense and nescience? Dis-association from the body, incoherence in the mind and dispossession of the soul keep us locked into the Borg delusion, spellbound to an obsolete divide and conquer civilization. To free ourselves from the sacrilege of Thanatos we must steep ourselves in the notion of first doing no harm, plus grok the absolute conscionablity of The Golden Rule. Real change requires that we grant ourselves unconditional original blessing and release everything that doesn't bless us and that isn't aligned with our highest wellbeing. Then we can offer that same magnanimous presence and clear vote of acceptance, allegiance and assurance to others.

In a competitive, violent culture we learn how to repress emotion, with thought, muscles and substances. Thus we lose our inner guide, our voice of Godspeak, our connection to the earth and Kosmos. This divorce from our inner being creates a peripheral narcissistic culture in which this dissociation process increases till all meaning and value is lost, all depth is lost. This is a dangerous condition for there is a pathological loss of "care" over what happens. We are cut off from the nobility of the past and the vision for the future, and try to make up for the loss of soul in substitute gratifications that weaken our condition still further. Clarity is achieved in the still point between opposites. Thus we cannot be at peace or at home in our flesh while there is conflict and competition between the poles, charges, hemispheres and sexes.

Love, or the music of the spheres, is the binding force of spin that forms and informs matter. This exquisite resonance of increasing order and complexity, is the genesis of the Universe unfolding in infinite perfection. In the human body love builds energy through the expansion of the synchrotronic heartfield, which imparts greater spin to the body's atoms allowing for the transmutation of the elements and an increase in exotic matter on which the life-blueprint is established. By increasing heart expansion we increase the **Orbitally Rearranged Monatomic Elements** (ORMEs) through which our soul superconducts the information for constructing the liquid crystal form of the body and the highest, subtle and causal levels of the spectrum of consciousness. Thus the greater the heart expansion in a raw-remineralized body the greater the potential for reaching translucent, transparent, multiperspective, Timeless levels of consciousness (ie: cosmic consciousness) via superluminal integration. The more ORMEs we have in our bodies and environment, the higher our kundalini, the higher our kundalini the more ORMEs created in the body.

High spin efficiency requires "high energy" and "low noise," therefore abundant ATP production in a body with low inflammation and free radical oxidation is essential to reach the more elevated states of HUman consciousness. Cosmic consciousness emerges from the vacuum flux or Zeropoint driven by the central point of the vector equilibrium between the opposite spins of the poles, charges and sexes. Thus the more perfect our spin, the higher the capacity of our atoms to maintain their integrity against free radical decay and "disintegration," and the greater our potential to tap into the Unified Field of cosmic consciousness. Without high spin and the plugging into Zeropoint the intellect even when primed for the Good, is ineffectual at the causal level on earth. Thus the Flatland or Hindbrain human with all his power still feels powerless to effect change. The sense of being out of control due to atomic dissonance forces the individual to compensate by trying to control others, the world and their fate. Through raising our spin, quietening our "noise" and delving into the still-point we learn to comply and cooperate with the Universal Flow and surrender to the All, and not the delusional errant ways of fallen man out of sync with the evolutionary upliftment of life.

The Universe dreams us and we are lived by the universe and thus full surrender and receptivity to the central fulcrum of Zeropoint permits full capacity and full effectuation, whereupon we become One with Universe as our bodymind and emotions are brought up to Universal or causal speed. In a culture afraid of emotion and feeling this holds us back in the brain retarded shadow zone, unable to build the energy and heart expansion necessary for reaching transcendent levels. Emotion freely flowing and fully lived is the river that binds the individual, the culture, the Earthsoul and God in a synthesis of our highest synergetic potential. Alchemical death and resurrection is necessary to throw off the mortal armored skin of the Borg whereupon spin can quicken for cosmic level initiation. The Good (God), or love, is the unifying music that creates greater integration and the full actualization of our epic destiny. We discover our rightful place in the whole by widening our circle of compassion to embrace all living creatures and the whole of nature and its beauty.

A kundalini awakening is simply the amplification of the play of the poles, charges, hemispheres and sexes—the energy that drives the Kosmos itself.

I am fascinated with the central point in the middle of the gyro for you can see how the twisting of spacetime down into infinite compression creates gravity. Fascinating too how spin relates to levels of consciousness and how higher levels tap deeper into transpersonal omniscience through the nexus point between opposite spins. In this sense you can begin to view the power and faculty of advanced beings in a new light. Due to the high spin the Presence of a mystic, saint or yogi alters the spacetime around themselves which others can "feel." Whereas someone of feeble consciousness, low energy/spin and who is sick or toxic—that is a living crystal that is malformed—you can feel their insubstantial gravity well as weak, warped or irritating, and observe that their subjectivity is narcissistic, myopic and self-serving, ie: non-radiant. The high spin state is the secret to thriving because it permits us to witness from the all seeing Eye of Horus in clarity, purity, precision, presence, providence and OM-power.

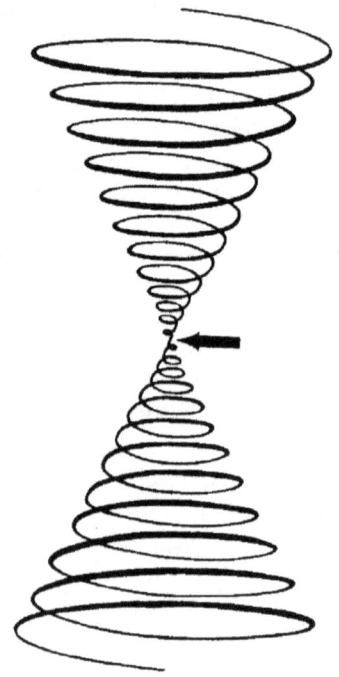

Words used to describe the mystic apprehension of central axis of opposing vortices through which the universe autopoetically self-organizes are: *Balance, vector equilibrium, maximum coherency, eye of the hurricane, singularity, pivot, fulcrum, still-point, silence, phase conjugation, conjunction, infinite density, maximum compression, omni-dimensional, neutral resting state, relaxation, love-trust, Samadhi, Flow, the Zone…Christ (crucifix), Grokking and Enlightenment.*

METHODS OF INCREASING MENTAL CLARITY

Fasting increases mental clarity through reducing the "noise" produced by toxicity, blockage, mucus, depolarization and metabolic inefficiency. Increasing oxygen, exercise, breathing, hydrogen peroxide, structured water and alkalinizing pH diet, chlorophyll from remineralized green plants decreases brain fog, as does all other methods of increasing O_2. Germanium is a trace mineral that increases O_2 and improves immunity. Germanium occurs in high amounts in many healing plants such as garlic, aloe, comfrey, chlorella, ginseng, the shitake mushroom, & watercress. Other things that reduce the "noise" of brain fog include grounding, sungazing and sunbathing, soaking in Nature's frequencies, negative ions, overcoming insulin resistance, removing transfats and other damaged fats from the diet, avoiding cooked food especially cereals/dairy/processed foods, and establishing an anti-candida diet.

Adopt a raw diet filled with chlorophyll, papaya and goji berries for betacarotene, colorful plant pigments and phytonutrient rich colorful raw foods. Beet juice can open up blood vessels and increase blood flow/oxygen to a critical region of the brain. Vinpocetine and Ginkgo—increases blood flow to the brain, hence oxygenates your brain cells. Oxygen, movement, exercise, grounding, sunshine, mindful sleep, friendships and meaningful work are very important to brain function. Lecithin has specifically been found to be ineffective at treating dementia, while Alpha GPC is 40% choline by weight and is able to cross the blood brain barrier intact.

Chelating heavy metals with **niacin, ribose and EDTA** in capsules (in quantities in which the niacin flush is "just" palpable) is an effective way of removing calcium deposits, reducing free radicals and raising ATP production necessary for consciousness. Highly detoxing (methylating) plants such as garlic mustard (cruciferous) and heavy metal chelators such as celentro and blue green algae help reinstate receptor efficiency. Nootropics, Folic acid, pantethine, Bcomplex, sublingual B12, Alpha lipoic, L-carnitine, Vitamin C around 8000 mg/day, liposomal Vitamin C, lecithin and Omega-3 sources and Taurine for neuroinhibition. Ginger tea, raw ginger beer from ginger root and lemon juice will reduce inflammation and settle the stomach brain. Rub rosemary essential oil into shins, jaw and temples. By mixing Mucuna, Caapi and Gingko and taking around: 2 x 000 capsules I was able to integrate the bliss of kundalini, come out of brain fog and achieve a newfound lucidity.

OTHER NOOTROPICS: L-Pyroglutamic Acid, Coenzyme Q10, N-acetyl cysteine (NAC), Agmatine Sulfate, Glutathione, Carnosine, Phenylalanine, Taurine, Arginine, Trimethylglycine, Tyrosine, DHA-Omega-3, DHEA, DMAE and Centrophenoxine, NADH, Piracetam, Noopept, Theanine, Huperzine, Vinpocetine, Pyroglutamate, Acetyl L-carnitine and L, Lysine, Ribose, Phosphatidylserine, Sunflower Lecithin, Spirulina, Vitamin C, Magnesium Ascorbate, Chaga, Artichoke. Plus 2 B-Complex a day. Mucuna can be mixed with MAO inhibiting Banisteriopsis caapi and Bacopa for stressful days. Lion's mane mushroom, psilocybin mushroom and niacin was recommended by Paul Stamets for increasing creative genius. Sex hormone potency IS life potency and the power to effect change in accord with the dictates of Eros.

HOW TO SPARK OFF KUNDALINI

The peak experience of kundalini awakening allows participation in the World-brain/ Earth-soul, through the dysidentification with the conditioned stage that we are at. Our kundalini awakening will arise in direct relation to the specific armor/archetype that we have constructed.

Kundalini is the transconscious Master, only she knows what she is doing. To rise to the grace of the Master we must work on regenerating, revitalizing, reenzyming, detoxing, remineralizing, opening the body and getting out of the way of her supreme counsel and direction. Transmutation IS us, when we stop being a errant mutant. Metamorphosis "includes" purification but it is actually much, much more than that. Purification is simply the function of clearing stuff out of the way that is interfering with the building of a higher temple of the body to house the deeper degree of spirit. The flow of consciousness in the body, that is self-communication, is a matter of the amount of energy times conductivity divided by resistance.

When we raise Kundalni we are essentially raising the Lifeforce by making the physical cells strong enough to endure the energy and light of consciousness. The cooked food Western body is weak and inflammatory and generally not strong enough to handle kundalini without creating tissue damage from glycation, oxidation, catabolysis and nerve damage. For this reason I don't advise anyone to set about with the intention of raising kundalini—alternatively I suggest they focus on detoxification, remineralization, earthing/grounding, sun meditation, increasing the % of raw in diet, exercise, hanging, breathing, giving your greatest gift, following the muse etc....

Fortunately for them most cooked-fooders will not awaken in their lifetime due to the lack of cellular energy (ATP) and enzyme charge, and to occlusion of the light by plaques caused by ama, toxicity, and the blockage of cell membranes etc... In a cooked body there are simply inadequate resources to break through the metabolic refuse and barricades to consciousness (Spirit) in order for kundalini to become initiated. Rather than focusing on trying to awaken kundalini we should be fixing the main factors leading to the modern western cooked body being inappropriate for awakening. When looking at why humans are the most unhealthy species one has to consider the elements missing in our diet from demineralization, human food production and cooking methods and compare that with a primate diet in the wild, then we see we are missing Omega-3, magnesium (greens), silicon, B17 and huge amounts of vitamin C and wild phytochemicals.

• RAISING

Simply changing to a raw diet will spark off kundalini (David Wolfe); keeping the blood charged with alkaline minerals from raw vegetables, and adopting an antioxidant rich diet to prevent nerve and cell membrane damage. Sprouted greens and green smoothies remove energy blocks allowing repressions to loosen their hold. DHEA, ginseng and other sex hormone enhancers, romantic love and frequent exposure to unique, authentic people, places and experiences maintains our enthusiasm for life. The fastest method of raising kundalini is sungazing meditation on the rising or setting sun for 15-30 minutes/day. Other initiatory practices that fuel the chi flame are fasting, **alternating hot & cold**, that is plunging temperature changes such as sauna, cold shower, or nude-sunbathing then jumping in cold water. To open and get energy flowing you can use movement and vibration such as binaural music, toning, mantra, singing, hanging, running and some stretching like yoga, meditation, breath of fire, holotropic breathing, trance dancing, drumming, Guru devotion and shaktipat, camping in nature, ocean sailing, and shamanic journeying.

• ADAPTATION

Thus once kundalini is initiated and active avoid sustained meditation that "lasers" consciousness in any one place such as the third eye and adopt energy integrating-movement meditations like the Taoist microcosmic orbit. The theory behind this caution is that to continue to fire up the "spark plugs" once the engine is already going will burn the body out faster than it can sufficiently recuperate. Adaptive-integrative practices are those that help to integrate energy, cleanse, ground, stabilize the body and mind and fortify the cells. You will need a get regular cardio exercise like running and some kind of energy movement work like Reiki or Qi gong (Mantak Chi). For blockages to energy the main thing we need to address is numbness, and the underlying muscle contraction underneath the numbness; stimulating nerve flow using touch, bodywork, holding, tapping, shaking, rebounding, hot and cold, mud baths, grounding in nature. Reconnect by camping out under the stars, vision quests, sweat-lodges, mineral pools, exercising in nature, peer companionship and the Inner Arts, in nature. To establish the growth or healing frequencies, the is the fastest way to actively turn off the flight-flight response and turn on the parasympathetic vagus nerve is sex, the Inner Arts and meditation.

• DEALING WITH ACUTE KUNDALINI SYNDROME

If you are experiencing difficult symptoms you need to build up that organ or function, not suppress the symptoms. Most negative symptoms are due to toxicity, deficiency and cooked-culture weakly built tissues, stagnation and lack of exercise, plus separation from nature's energies. Use the water and earth to calm the fire. Lie on the grass for as many hours it takes to "normalize" and put your left face on the grass as well. Go barefoot and wear natural fiber clothing as much as possible. If you are near clean ocean, streams or lakes use that water to sit and swim in and bury yourself in the sand to ground out the kundalini heat. Drink more water than usual as the amplified prana will dehydrate you, and eat the most colorful raw fruit and vegetables you can find in small amounts throughout the day, like a grazing animal.

The facial distortion (similar to stroke victims) on the left side does eventually go away once the left side of the body returns to its more regular electromagnetic flux, it can take years for the face to get completely symmetrical again, so don't worry about it. Inquire into what your body is telling you to do. If you feel you are being pulled down into the ground then lie on the ground until your body is satisfied, this normally takes at least half an hour. If you feel drawn to be outside then change your lifestyle to incorporate outside living and long walks. Try and use the energy creatively and productively in whatever form its seems to emerge in words, ideas, artwork, music etc... But if divine mandate or Muse-vocation is forthcoming don't force it, as you are already undergoing the most extreme "work" — the alchemical transmutation of the flesh.

Once you are already initiated generally stay away from spiritual groups and gurus and develop your own practice of integrating the energy. Play with children, animals, do gardening and crafts etc... The reason for this is that when you are already in overwhelm, being around spiritually focused people could lead to psychosis unless they themselves have already gone through massive kundalini awakening and have rationally integrated the process. The symbolic, archetypal nature of religion is dangerous to the mind that has been wrenched open by kundalini fire and is having to process vastly increased data in the form of psychic, gnostic, sensory, temporal and biophysical information.

Long walks of up to 5 hours a day is how I maintained my sanity. You cannot rely on regular society for help, comfort or solace as non-initiated people can be unhealthy to interact with, for the "blockages" in people are triggered by your heightened fire and they often act out their dark nature, or conversely if they are "clear" they will be stimulated into greater angelic mode by your energy. I know it is hard…the hardest thing you have ever done, but be grateful that this is happening to you…so few humans ever get to experience what you are going through.

Basically when you increase the cell voltage and the light through an inflammatory body with incoherent structures, weak hydrogen/water bonding and inadequate reserves — you increase oxidation, glycation, flocculation, rancidity, aging, inflammation, dehydration and mutation, which creates a catabolic breakdown of tissues and molecules. The body thus basically eats itself and will transform and rebuild itself if given the time, space, frequencies and resources to do so.

The greater the light flow, the greater the catabolic breakdown during the metamorphosis, thus if you fight the breakdown, dieoff and collapse and don't give the bodymind what it needs for transmutation you will not be transformed, merely translated into a dislocated, displaced slightly awake Borg. This under-achieved enlightenment is FAR WORSE than never having been initiated in the first place. For then we are caught permanently in limbo between being in awake-heaven and unconscious-hell.

Thrival necessitates a reduction in fear and neurosis, thus the weak reactive ego has to progressively die within the social crisis and cultural upheaval. We are undergoing a restitutional crisis of waking up to what we should have been doing all along. Thus our moral conscience is catching up with the rest of our development, providing the solid foundations for a vastly superior future. Focusing on personal spirituality at the expense of efforts toward creating the new civilization is idle escapism. Planting trees, for example, is a healthier more honorable form of meditation than is sitting on a cushion.

Things are changing rapidly now, we need to figure out where we fit in and jump into the fast moving stream. We shouldn't fear the pace of change, for this speed is releasing us from a past which is no longer working for us.

The sooner we let go of the immaturity and moral bankruptcy of the Borg, the faster the new way comes into being. Certainty on doing the "right thing" and remaining true to the Muse will carry us through. The Muse doesn't arise within a vacuum, it needs social, artistic and scientific information and stimulation. So wherever and whatever you are called to feed the Muse, do that. Go on adventures, risk, try new things, new places, new people. Ask where you can best serve in both immediately and in the long-term and then work with efficacy towards that.

To overcome our normal body dissociation and numbness we need to grow "ears" in every cell of our body. As we employ this cellular listening as a daily practice we progressively soften the feeling-sense or sensualization of the body, building the skill to receive ever more subtle nuanced information, and incorporate complexity and paradox. When we address sovereignty at the biochemical level besides the neurotransmitter precursor amino acids and cofactors we can work towards generating full sovereign strength, focus and endurance, plus establish a lifestyle protocol for increasing receptor sensitivity, VO_2 Max, mitochondrial optimization, remineralization, and hormone/neurotransmitter potency.

• MAINTAIN A HEALTHY NERVOUS SYSTEM

You are as sovereign and emancipated as your nervous system is strong. Psychopathy, delusion and crimes against nature only occur when the hardware for consciousness has been compromised by generations of toxicity, trauma and anti-life living. It is so important to ensure optimal nutrition for your nervous system that I will include the following nerve sheath information in the Inner Arts book, because there is not much point doing inner exercises when our metabolic and physical machinery is weak and impaired. If the nerve damage is degenerative, heavy metals may be involved, which would necessitate a *chelation diet*. Difficult symptoms and ill health are a sign of inferior subatomic, molecular, cellular, neurological, EMF and light connection. Improve the bodymind structure, function and communication and what you experience as demons, transform to the lightside and become the daemon, the Muse, the Holy Spirit or Presence.

• CALM FORMULA

This calms and balances the central nervous system without exacerbating the kundalini symptoms. Good for reducing the hyperactivation of the sympathetic nervous system during kundalini peak and the associated hypertension and insomnia. It calms one all day, reduces mental "noise," without tiring or reducing intelligence. Good for ADHD, panic attacks, anxiety and depression as well. Mix powders together, rebottle and keep in the fridge. Take up to 1 teaspoon in a glass of water on an empty stomach first thing in the morning half an hour before eating, and again before sleep. Take 1 B Complex along with this formula. *The follow quantities can be purchased from beyond-a-century. com* 5 http (L-tryptophan), 20 gms; L-Glutamine, 300 gm; DL Phenylalanine 100gm; Calcium-Magnesium, 8 oz; Vitamin C/Ascorbic Acid Powder, 300gm.

• NERVE SHEATHS

Silicon from Horsetail tea, Cornsilk, or Nettle. Nerve sheaths—lecithin, B-complex (B12, Folic acid), Oceanic ORMUS, Multi-mineral, Shilajit Mineral, Kelp, Irish moss, Dulse, Fulvic Acid, Vitamin D3, **Olive leaf, Rhodiola, Gingko,** Frankincense, Amla, Kiwifruit, Gooseberries, Camu camu, Fish, Nuts, Cacao, Avocados, Sprouted Legumes, Spinach, Lambsquarters, Nettles, Horsetail, Watercress, Alfalfa, Red Clover, Anthocyanidin Flavonoids in all berries including Elderberries and Mulberries, Ginseng, Hawthorn Berry, Bromelain, Guggul, Frankincense, Licorice Root, **Lion's Mane Mushroom**, Astragalus, Bacopa, Turmeric, Ginger Root, Cinnamon, Grapeseed and/or Pinebark extract. Omega-3 is needed for the cardiolipin lining of the mitochondria, and when Omega-3 levels are low the mitochondria are probably burning dirty and creating more free radicals. So you need to increase your plant colors, Vitamin C, Alpha Lipoic and other antioxidants when increasing Omega-3. Wild salmon; Krill oil is better than fish oil, because the high levels of natural antioxidants in Krill prevent the oil from going rancid. Spirulina and plant sources are better than fish oil which is already rancid. Plant sources include moringa leaf, purslane, and the seeds/oils of hemp, flax, chia, Kiwi fruit, Pomegranate, Perilla, Walnuts, Sacha Inchi, camu camu, and borage, spirulina and other bluegreen algae. Other oils for strong nerves include Black currant oil, Borage oil and Evening primrose oil, Olive leaf oil, Raw coconut oil, Ratfish oil, Avocado oil, Grapeseed oil, Oregano oil, Sea Buckthorn Oil, Blackseed Oil, Rosemary oil, Helichrysum essential oil.

• CHELATION OF HEAVY METALS & RADIONUCLIDES

It is important to consider that toxins in the body have an accumulative, synergistic negative effect thus, it is vital to cleanse the system of heavy metals along with radionuclides. Heavy metals set up conditions that lead to inflammation in arterial walls, joints and tissues, causing more calcium to be drawn to the area as a buffer. Medical chelation is done to reduce calcium plaques on arterial walls using a synthetic amino acid EDTA (ethylene diamine tetraacetic acid). Oral chelation works best through the synergistic effect of combining EDTA, niacin, & ribose with other natural chelating agents. **Heavy Metal Removing Chelation Foods And Supplements:**
Ashitaba, Green tea, Chlorella, Cilantro, Parsley, Nettle, Ginkgo biloba, Red ginseng extract, Green tea extract, Aloe gel, Olive leaf, Water melon juice, Banana stem juice, whole pumpkin juice with skin and seeds, Hawthorn berry, Cayenne, Pine Bark extract, Grape seed extract and Grape skin extract. Vitamin E and D, Quercetin, CoQ10, Vitamin C, Beta-carotene and all antioxidants. Magnesium, Sodium alginate, Selenium, Silicon and Zinc gluconate. Vitamin B's such as folic acid, inositol, choline and niacinamide 400-500 mg of each daily. Amino acids: L-cysteine, L-glutathione, Methionine, Lysine, Proline, L-taurine, N-acetyl cysteine, L-Carnosine and Selenomethionine. L-lysine is an amino acid involved in the structural repair of damaged blood vessels. It has a beneficial effect on lead toxicity and high blood pressure. To increase liver detoxification add Milk thistle, Dandelion root, Schizandra and 6000 mg of vitamin C per day along with bioflavonoids and Alpha Lipoic Acid to promote liver activity.

Kelp contains a powerful chelating agent called Mannitol. The algaes spirulina or chlorella are needed to bind up the liberated heavy metals to carry them out of the body. Rice bran chelates reactive iron. Russian black radish, MSM, the cabbage family, garlic, and garlic mustard are sources of sulfur, which binds with copper and other heavy metals so they can be eliminated, and many heavy metal binding proteins contain sulfur. Sulfur is also important for liver detoxification. Activated Clays (Zeolite and Fulvic acid), bentonite clay, apple pectin and charcoal. Plant-based enzymes (bromelain, lipase, catalase) can be added to ensure optimal utilization of all of the above nutrients and assist in the breakdown and removal of plaques. A pesto of soaked raw pumpkin seeds and cilantro is a standard in the chelation diet, as are all colorful fruits and vegetables, raw juices and sprouts.

• RADIATION PROTECTION

Radiation mitigation requires methylation (sulfur binding of toxins), antioxidants and reducing the body's toxic load. Astaxanthin, Ashitaba, Aloe Vera, Chamomile, Chaparral, Echinacea, Garlic Mustard, Olive leaf, Neem, Ginkgo, Uva Ursi, Yucca Root, Noni Fruit & Seed, Jojoba, Juniper, Turmeric, Graviola, Frankincense, Myrrh, Reishi Mushroom, Niacin, Cysteine, Bentonite clay, Zeolites, Fulvic Acid, Pyrophyllite clay, Activated charcoal. Bladderwrack, Kelp, chlorella, spirulina, dulse and nori as well as miso broth. Adopt a mineral rich diet (natural iodine Lugol's solution, iron, B-12, ginseng, selenium, boron, & zinc). For methylation eat sulfur-rich vegetables of the cabbage family: garlic mustard, kale, watercress, Brussel sprouts, turnips, cauliflower, arugula, mustard greens, bok choy, swiss chard, onions, garlic, (MSM).

Increase antioxidant rich berries of all kinds, kale, spinach, plums, oranges, red grapes, red bell pepper, cherries, eggplant, lime juice, colorful root veges & carrots. Increase beta carotene: papaya, goji, spinach, carrots, yams, squash, pumpkin, and beets. Reduce sugar/carb/grain consumption to bare minimum and focus on seeds, nuts, sprouts, green and living foods and living water. Epsom salts, sea salt and baking soda and borax baths to help pull out the radiation from your body. Negative ions draw out radiation, hydrate cells, flush toxins, hence the need for grounding and nature. Probiotics are essential to a radioprotective diet. In turn, prebiotics like pectin and inulin (chicory root, yucca, cassava root) are essential to the viability of probiotics, as they are food for the beneficial bacteria.

Incorporate high fiber for broom action in the GI tract to speed elimination of heavy metals use flaxseed, chia seed, ricebran and psyllium powder. The skin of fruits and vegetables are high, not only in pectin, but also in a wide range of antioxidants and other phytonutrients. The pith of the citrus contains about 30% pectin. Apple Pectin reduces Cesium-137 load by over 62% in one month and pectin is also a chelator of other positively charged heavy metals. Coconuts and coconut water are very high in potassium and magnesium. Potassium reduces uptake of cesium-137. Argan Oil and Carbon 60 protects skin from UV. http://gaeasgarden.com/c60.

END NOTE

ASCENT OF THE INNER MAN

Spirit is ceaselessly seeking to emerge through the obstruction that diverts its rainbow path.

We might propose that the ultimate root cause of false power and the pathological power pyramid is the chronic blockage, inhibition and damming-up of lifeforce, impulses and urges, which causes the constipation of consciousness and the backing up of metabolism into the Toxic Brain Syndrome. Unconscious to its own motivations Hindbrain culture therefore is plagued with the propagation of a hyperbolic swing between repression, perversion and explosion—an obvious bipolar pattern that prevents the long-term incremental sustainability of enculturation. It is obvious therefore that Borg civilization must periodically collapse under the weight of its own unhappy corruption and lack of emotional development.

The retardation of brain function within the shame/blame game leads to the sadomasochistic phenomena of conflict and war, which must then inevitably be enacted as a release for the constipation of toxic brain chemistry. This acting out of accumulated tension is a causal agent of violence even more so than for the common causes of war, namely territory, booty and defense. Recent rapid increases in the technology of war, have made assured mutual destruction inevitable, which essentially makes war obsolete.

If humanity evolved beyond the scarcity mentality of the Hindbrain to a post-egoic, mystic regenerous level then war would end immediately, because the causes for war would disappear. The answer therefore in creating a strong non-violent society is to train infant children in emotional intelligence and to express their truth more fluently, this will help to enhance their empathetic, affiliative capacity, ensuring they have the skills to meet their "higher" needs in a healthy way. By consciously facilitating the humanizing process the crippling descent into our lower nature need not become the law of the land and the height of misguided patriotism and accelerating evil.

"Man's eminence lies in his reason and in the power to think, which distinguishes him from all other living creatures. And man's reason teaches him that peaceful cooperation and collaboration under the division of labor is a more beneficial way to live than violent strife." Ludwig von Mises

The fallen state of humankind IS the sadomasochistic Hindbrain Borg, and it has been my job to "fix it" first within myself, and then to help reduce the suffering that the power-over domain inflicts on the human species and the world. My spiritual vocation started off in the 1980's when having sailed to Hawaii from New Zealand I was given the knowledge that full emotional integration is necessary for growth, evolution and the establishment of Truth.

It became apparent to me that the egoic, linguistic narrative self of the left-brain needed to reestablishing contact with the right-brain, heart and solar plexus intelligences.

Over the course of 30 years I have inspected the mechanisms of the fall of man and have come to an understanding of how the "rise of man" can be brought about. Understanding the neuroscience of sovereignty, along with the Inner Arts and spiritual nutrition shifts Borg recovery into a higher gear, from merely surviving and muddling through to becoming the absolute best version of ourselves. Since as a culture we have not consciously inspected the reasons for the descent of humanity nor rectified its causes, we are for all intents and purposes living in a socioeconomy of death and decline.

The human species is stuck in the arrested development of scarcity mentality, obsolescence and senescence, we are thus in the process of recycling ourself, which means there is more "profit" in death than in life. It is however only the Borg human that is succumbing to Thanatos, while the sovereign human is just starting to come into being. To move forward we have to create our own abundance systems separate from the mainstream economic system. Thus we have to be smart enough to use the existing economic system in order to get out of it. The sovereign human is Self-possessed and differentiated from the "context" of his or her anthropological conditions such that self-determinancy is not an option, it is an unavoidable necessity.

The Borg civilization is a cult or "consensus trance," and so in order to operate from Self-will and positive agency and to not be controlled by the automatic Borg default program, we must personally eliminate addictions and avoidance behaviors, dearmor, deprogram, question everything, Know Thyself, tune into our Daemon, get into spontaneous Flow, integrate body-mind-soul, and generate forward moving momentum. Adventure, new challenges, interhemispheric & bilateral movements, dexterity and coordination exercises, bodywork, hydrotherapy or any novel experience increases neurogenesis.

Family and culture are an apriori given context. We are programmed for good and bad by the time, place and sociosphere of our arrival on planet earth. We are an inevitable product of the family, culture and the times that made us. Our "job" as conscious sovereign beings is to refine the cultural conditions and social circumstances to that which serves higher HUman values, and to eliminate that which holds back the full flourishing of ourselves, our species and all life. To submit unquestionably to a culture of death is spiritual suicide, and a sad waste of unfathomable potential not yet born.

Physicist and author Leonard Mlodinow (www.projectimplicit.net) found that people are often not in control of their own judgments, perceptions, biases, beliefs and actions, which typically come from the brainwashing of stereotypes in the media that have entered the subconscious and act subliminally on how the unconscious mind shapes our experience of the world. Conscious/unconscious divergences reflect the split-mindedness of the Borg that has to repress a vast percentage of full HUman awareness in order to submit to the constant *Self versus World* dilemmas and doublebinds of this anti-HUman society. Such self-deception and resistance to Reality constitutes the fallen state of Man. Essentially gooing up the works of human intercourse with Reality. A state of both conscious non-responsiveness and subliminal nescience serves the survival of the slave, while preventing the emergence of the noble sovereign or mystic.

The sovereign gains social resilience and emotional regulation by establishing a high-energy lifestyle, and detoxifying and dearmoring the bodymind. By raising our own frequency we produce the set, setting and atomic structure for a positive experience of life that generates the positive emotion and propagates an ongoing positive experience of life. To thrive the sovereign must renegotiate all social contracts to fit a world of self-responsibility and freedom, where all individuals reside in the unequivocal equity of Source. Respecting the sovereignty and divinity of all living things determines the quality of our emotions and our subsequent behaviors and adaptations.

Wholeness is our native state, and so all that separates us from our daemonic self, holds us suspended and stagnated in our demonic self. Growth is a detox process requiring deprogramming of the conditioning that creates and maintains the ego-armor. Thus in order to grow we must eliminate mistaken ideas, beliefs, self-images, reactions and behaviors that shackle us to a crippled deformed figment of our true nature. The return to unity with the Cosmos is possible to any individual who is willing to recognize that his true home is to be found by turning within and correcting his perception and feeling, and changing his relationship to the All.

Since our mind works on three levels: the conscious, of which we are aware, and the subconscious and transconscious that is hidden from us, we must cultivate our life like a garden, covering all aspects of the growth and creativity cycle to ensure physical, emotional, mental and spiritual uplift. The automatic **subliminal nature of cultural enslavement** means that we are not aware of our own higher HUmanity, nor are we conscious of the parameters of our cage. The Given default nature of the cultural context of our lives subliminally affects our judgments, perceptions, biases, beliefs and actions. To become aware of the cultural context and our place in the continuum frees up our ability to be self-determinate.

Negativity is a "choice" to negate sovereignty or empowerment by tuning the dial towards the courser emotions. If humanity has been in the grip of negative energy since the antediluvian age, then this is a self-administered funk. In order to change we must take total responsibility for where we have been and where we are going. The inability to FACE reality of negativity and shadow pushes it under the rug of a forced, desperate and immature positivism. Of course there is little growth, and a lot of the projection of evil and blame generated by taking such a casual and irresponsible stance to life. The negative is not to be indulged in, it is to be learned from and thereby contribute vital information for "course correction" and rectification.

Sublime objectivity or Fair Witnessing includes the light and the dark as two halves of the whole. Discursive thinking is simply ego validating itself, solidifying itself in a subject-object dance that creates a sense of identity in a body-mind, and a feeling of centrality at a superficial level. We tend to deny, disown and repress our negative internal feelings, and project them onto others. Thus other people mirror back to us our hidden emotions and feelings, which allows us to recognize and reclaim them.

Negative emotions are rampant within the sadomasochistic, power-mad, exploitative usury-civilization. Such social conditions breed constant inner conflict largely as a consequence of competition and insecurity such as - feeling fear, guilt, shame, fear of responsibility, jealousy, rebellion, sadness, anger, hopelessness, depression, criticism or other uncomfortable shadow emotions. This then leads to over-compensatory and avoidance behaviors such as self/other abuse, bullying, addiction, escapism, hoarding, conformity, anti-creativity, workaholism, isolation, pharmaceuticals, videogames, junk food and sedentarism etc...

Emotions and their environmental context are intrinsically bound in an infinite möbius strip of cause and effect. Acknowledging the complexity of the light and dark of life is important to psychological well-being. Negative emotions may also aid in our survival by providing cues that a health issue, relationship or other important matter needs our attention. Eudaemonic approaches to mental health and personal growth emphasize making sense of life's ups and downs by evaluating our experiences to discover meaning and self-understanding. Eudaemonic – means producing happiness and well-being: based on the idea that happiness is the outcome of proper conduct.

We kill what is HUman in us in order to submit to dehumanizing conditions. To succumb to scarcity mentality and avoid refining our being within the "liberties" of the true creative power of our unique cosmic being – is to miss out on the opportunity to be truly HUman within our own lifetime, and forgo the untold mystery, awe and power from fully incarnating our soul. There is no greater pleasure than apotheosis, or incarnating our soul, and yet the Borg spends 100% of its efforts avoiding such an immediate, eternal and obvious process. Instead of backing away from negative emotions, the sovereign accepts them and turns to confront life's adversities, and in the process establishes greater clarity to proceed down the path of goal fulfillment.

Serious investigation of the shadow (conflicts/blocks/voids) within helps us to see the light. If we are deeply aware of happenstance we will notice that if we go too far in one direction and become unbalanced, the universe will constantly persuade us back to go in the opposite direction again. If our nervous system is shot from bad habits, accumulated stress and beliefs that hurt and diminish us, then we can only give what we ARE to the world. Pain and difficult emotions are essentially there to protect our sovereign center (higher self). However they can be hijacked and used for all manner of nefarious purposes, but basically our emotional body is in a sense more truthful and divine than our minds if only we could read its meaning.

It is just that in a repressive, emotionally sick society we have not learnt to process, integrate, sort out, assimilate, and detoxify from all our emotions. The power-driven cultural structure makes for a retarded and aborted emotional realm, and it is this, plus the degradation of our physical form itself, which is largely holding back the human species in its delinquent-animalistic (distressed) form. This is also the reason why we are morally off the rails as a species, for we cannot "hear" our higher self, because of all the noise from the sewage of mal-digested emotions. Light is the catalyst for darkness to evolve, and darkness is the catalyst for Light to evolve.

The whole HUman naturally responds to cosmic order, Universal Law, gnostic guidance and biological navigation without having to be taught or controlled by punishment and reward. The compartmentalized, broken human (the Borg) does not Know Thyself, and doesn't know that it doesn't know. The lack of Phi coherency that we have inflicted on our environment, food and body, locks us into a perpetually cosmically disconnected state. Whereas sovereignty is the path to rectify this dissociation and reclaim the whole HUman—to reconstruct the cosmic alignment from soil to soul.

Understanding that the "noise" of the discombobulated self is not who we really are leads us to propose the big question—"Just who and what are we?" If we are at all interested in experiencing ourself as a HUman, we will naturally gravitate towards the alignment with our sovereign center. The convergence of our multidimensional composite self on the Heart's true calling to Know Thyself is geometrically progressive once the first intuition and steps are taken. The Solar Heart is the nondual connection to the Universe through its power to remain open in the face of darkness due to the radiant quality of coherent light.

A human being is comprised of an ever-changing and mysterious interior and exterior universe that we all inhabit, *knowingly* or not. The genuine seeker is passionately desiring to resolve the self/world schism and come into Phi alignment with the cosmos. The true heart desires to feel into reality, in order to discover or manifest an authentic Self—thus removing the sense of separation, to feel fully at home in the body on earth. The desire to really "Know Thyself," and to not be a mere hodgepodge of chemical responses to The Given chessboard, is our committed course correction to the Force of Eros, the creatrix of the Universe herself.

In the domain of neuroscience, executive power has been viewed as a function of the prefrontal cortex, which receives (monitors) sensory signals from other cortical regions and through feedback loops implements control. We evolve from where we are to where we want to be via "**metacognition**," or "the cognition about cognition," or "knowing about knowing." That is, being aware of and having conscious control over our own cognition and monitoring our progress towards desired goals. Metacognition refers to a level of thinking that involves active control over the thought process in learning situations, identifying strengths and weaknesses and adjusting their strategies to achieve favorable outcomes.

It is our choice whether we want to live in the death-culture, cooked, GMO, criminal medicine, obese, Metabolic X and mentally deranged world? Or whether we want to live in the enlightened, progressive, raw, permacultural, regenerative, anti-pharma, remineralized and reforested world? By our actions we shall know ourselves!

True science is found in the spaces where the old science doesn't fit.

THE DIVIDED BRAIN AND HINDBRAIN SOCIETY

What trigger in the brain causes people to break from habit and routine? Neurons in the posterior cingulate cortex (PCC) in the central-back region of the brain ramp up firing rates and peak just before a divergent behavior occurs. This spike in "activation energy" in the brain leads to the divergent thinking and a change in the course of action because of it. The proximity of the agentic "change course" area of the brain to the discriminatory "judicial center" of the brain...comprising at it were the *posterior cingulate cortex* and the *anterior cingulate cortex*, suggests to me that our sense of morality, righteousness, fairness and wholeness is intimately related to whether we tend to become paralyzed, stagnant and risk avoidant, or whether we feel free, strong, capable and able enough to chart our own course. The posterior cingulate cortex must reach "activation energy" in order for us to change our circumstances as we feel fit...in order to experience feeling fully alive.

By reducing oxygen via narrowing the blood supply caffeine shuts down the prefrontal cortex and the posterior cingulate cortex, while activating the limbic system and visual cortex. Alcohol similarly numbs regions of the brain needed for sovereign, agentic and creative will. Inter-hemispheric communication is key to creativity, risk assessment and beneficiary change. If we are too awake for our social environment we become the black sheep or outsider in our family, community or workplace. Hindbrain individuals may spread malicious gossip about us, concoct lies, insult us, give the evil eye and strive to obtain dopamine fixes through devious means so that they feel less threatened by our penetrating consciousness, or apparent moral-superiority. This is the basis for the Tall Poppy Syndrome, and the situation where the crabs in the bucket pull escaping crabs back down into the bucket in an attempt to save themselves from their captivity -. leading to no crabs escaping.

If we do not stand up to malicious rumors, false accusations, gender harassment, sexual shaming, sexual competition, the usury of witches, and exploitative workplaces etc... then our sense of "fairness" is compromised... and our aggravated judicial center (*anterior cingulate cortex*) then interferes with the smooth functioning of the posterior part of the cingulate cortex that governs our capacity for "choice" and change. We can thus see how Hindbrain society maintains its customs of undermining the sovereignty, freedom, creativity and spiritual development of its citizens - by brain damaging their capacity for unique choice through systemic emotional and psychological abuse, financial inequity (unfairness) and sexual/gender harassment and exploitation.

In this way those that are most socially toxic (sociopaths) tend to rise to the top and capture the lives of slaves through brain damaging them and preventing their capacity to change, grow and become independent. Codependency and the accompanying borderline dissociative disorder is directly tied to the overworked and exhausted posterior and anterior cingulate cortexes... and the consequent disconnect between the two brain hemispheres...thereby reducing our capacity to be a whole, sovereign independent person...master of our world...and charting a sacred course into a transcendent future.

THE TRANSPERSONAL SELF

"Once we accept our limits, we go beyond them." Albert Einstein

The self-reflexive trait of "Theory of Mind" is the understanding the mind and the "mental world," giving us humans a multiperspectival view of "beliefs," plus the ability to penetrate the "maya of appearances," and the capacity for soul-searching and cogent introspection. As a characteristic of Theory of Mind "metacognition" can be defined as the process that reinforces one's subjective sense of being a self, thus we could called it "meta-subjectivity." As Socrates said "Know thyself." To go beyond yourself you must know yourself, but the greatest wisdom is in knowing that you know nothing.

Metacognition improves an individual's ability to understand their own mind and emotions compared to others. The sense of presence, or cognitive awareness and self-control diminishes worry, anxiety and existential dread. Meta-emotion or emotional-awareness, is the disciplined awareness of the cascading effect, the reactivity and blowback of our own emotions and those of others. In a presovereign group dynamic of emotional repression and disapproval based on systemic untruth, we learn to invalidate and dissociate from our own emotional intelligence, in which case we abort the spiritual development of the Frontopolar Cortex, the executive director of our will-power and our capacity to be HUman. Neglected prefrontal lobe development represents immaturity.

The principle area of the brain vital to the establishment of spiritual maturity or sovereignty is front-most part of the frontal lobe, "the Frontopolar Cortex." This Central Intelligence Area (CIA) that helps us predict future events from past experiences is more advanced in humans than other primates. The infantilism of the Borg is a psychosocial dis-ease caused by communal denial of emotional inter-subjectivity and loss of faith in our self-efficacy or ability to thrive caused by the neglected development of the spiritual executor — the Frontopolar Cortex. One of the definitions of sapience is "metacognition" or the detached ability to consciously think about thinking, giving us the ability to plan, check, monitor, select, revise, evaluate, and LEARN! Metacognition is central to developing differentiation, individuation, reciprocity, empathy, interdependence, self-regulation and sovereignty.

Periscopic thinking about the future engages the frontopolar cortex which then activates the medial prefrontal cortex or "Dorsolateral Cortex" that is active in enforcing will-power. The Frontopolar Cortex is therefore vital for intention, vision, delayed gratification, prioritization, resisting temptation, and overcoming automacy, reactivity and compulsion. In meditation, when we laser our mind on an area of our brain or body this acts to enliven, awaken, heal, integrate and evolve the form and function of that area. Thus by focusing on the brain area for future-sight we are able to grow the vision, and engage the will-power through which we may actively build a sovereign bodymind and establish a sovereign life

The great resolution, restitution and renaissance is upon us!.

APPENDIX A

VISIONARY & DREAM WORK

- Dreams often reveal to us the highest and deepest insights, and present us with a source of unlimited interest, wonder, creativity and psychic potential.
- Dreams need novel sensory and environmental input to produce more elaborate stories and scenes, because the brain is trying to adapt to new data and its mechanisms for processing novelty kick in producing more novelty.
- Fasting/detoxing produces deeper dreams and deeper life experience because it is one of the only things to clean cell receptors. High quality cedar essential oil will also clean synapses.
- Put on some music like Dreamtime by Steve Roach, or Awakened Mind #2 or Alpha/Delta and Theta wave binaural CD's Jeffrey Thompson
- A dab of Syrian rue-cinnamon oil under the ears and at the temples before bed helps to generate Alpha freqency for deeper more relaxed dreaming.
- Drink some high quality water and take 1 teaspoon of Magnesium ascorbate or Magnesium citrate before bed.
- Raw diet — increase energy conductivity and consciousness with enzymes, sprouts, raw juice, green smoothies.
- Green — regenerate with raw chlorophyll, remineralized soil, spirulina
- Sungazing — brain charging and defragging with photons, then moving into the dark.
- Nature — exposure to the elements for soul recharging and integration.
- Novelty — travel, the unknown, new experience and change increases neurogenesis.
- Visual Stimulation – nature, art, movies, computer animation, sacred geometry animations.
- Vision Quest — Questioning, surrender, exposure to the elements in nature.
- Relationships — Stimulating, meaningful, purposeful, creative
- Herbs — Valerian, Chamomile, Calea zacatechichi, Mugwort, Syrian rue, African dream herb (Entada rheedii/Silene capensis), Blue vervain, Skullcap
- Pyridoxine, B-6 enhances dream recall and vividness. Many of its activities are related to the metabolism of amino acids and other proteins including hemoglobin, serotonin, hormones, and prostaglandins.
- Sleep in complete darkness and take Melatonin before bed to increase the

vividness of dreams and improve the quality of sleep.
- Magnetic pillow (north pole), bed with head facing North
- 10-20 minutes of stretching, rolling on floor and massage prior to bed
- Deep breathing prior to sleep, or ozone foot bath to increase body oxygen.
- Toning—Huuu, Hmmm, Omm etc… Cleans the brain
- Dual-hemisphere—Dexterity Challenges, ambidextrous body movements
- Drumming, dancing, gardening, mud/clay baths, mineral pools, bodywork.

• DREAM HERBS
Borage, Nettle, St John's Wort, Mandrake, Mugwort – Artemisia vulgaris, Calea Zacatechichi was used by Mazatec shamans to induce vivid dreams, Entada rheedii, Silene capensis, Banisteriopsis caapi, Valerian boosts dream recall, Calamus root, Buchu, Bay Leaf, Marigold, Guayusa tea, Blue Vervain (used by Pawnee Indians), Morning Glory, Wood Betony, Wild Lettuce, California Poppy, Purslane, Blue Lotus, Holy Basil, Passionflower, Valerian, Chamomile. . Dragon's Blood (resin) is placed beneath the pillow to induce prophetic dreams, also burned to cause visions. Dragon's blood is often used to quicken and manifest intention. Hand rolled incense can be made with dragon's blood power and scotch.

• DREAM TEA TO SUP BEFORE SLEEP
Nettle, St John's Wort, Licorice, Ginger, Galangal, Orange Peel, Mugwort Mandrake, Calea Zacatechichi (used by Mazatec shamans to induce vivid dreams), Valerian, Fennel, Blue Vervain, Wild Lettuce, California Poppy, Hops. Galantamine, an extract of red spider lily induces more vivid dreaming

• SCENTS FOR DREAMING
Mugwort: Promotes lucid dreams, "astral travel" and visionary dreams. Contains thujone, the most active ingredient in absinthe.
Roman Chamomille: Calms dreams, reduces stress, and aids sleep. It is helpful for those who experience nightmares or restless sleep.
Lavender: Increases alpha waves, promoting tranquil, calm dreams. Relaxes the nervous system and reduces tension and irritability.
Rose: Works as an antidepressant. Promotes happy, pleasant dreams. Stimulating, uplifting, good as an antidote to sadness and fatigue.
To induce dreams of a prophetic nature, anoint your Third Eye chakra with Vervain juice or Vervain essential oil on a night of the full moon. Close your eyes, open your mind, and allow yourself to drift off to sleep.

• INSOMNIA

If you work with nature and her rhythms you will get your natural sleep back. The bright light of a computer can burn up your melatonin levels if you spend too much time in front of one. Don't spend more than 5 hours on your computer each day. Alkalinize your pH with raw-vege juice, raw-greens and conscious breathing. Massage your scalp before bed to release endorphins and serotonin. Also before be take melatonin, chamomile tea, Epsom salts baths and footbaths, magnesium, and topical magnesium on the back of the neck. Foods that contain melatonin are: Mustard seeds, almonds, sunflower seeds, cherries, flax seed, oats, rice, red radishes, poppy seeds, tomatoes and bananas. Vitamin B5 is a coenzyme acid that is essential for the synthesis of melatonin.

The amino acid Tryptophan is the precursor to Serotonin, an inhibitory neurotransmitter needed for sleep and relaxation. It calms, elevates pain threshold, promotes sleep and feeling of well being, reduces aggression and compulsive behavior. Tryptophan also stimulates Growth Hormone Release and relaxes the heart muscle and mind. Food sources of tryptophan include wild meat, dairy products, nuts, sunflower and sesame seeds, legumes, soybeans, broccoli, spinach, bananas, tuna, shellfish, seaweed, and turkey.

Vitamin B3 inhibits liver tryptophan pyrrolase and B3 also activates the enzyme that converts tryptophan to 5HTP. Thus taking 100mg B3 several times daily with meals will also serve to enhance the effectiveness of low-moderate tryptophan doses. Taking 50mg vitamin B6 once or twice daily with meals will also augment tryptophan-serotonin conversion, since B6 activates the decarboxylase enzyme that converts 5HTP to serotonin. Melatonin actually promotes increased brain serotonin through its ability to reduce cortisol levels, and reduced cortisol levels will lessen the activity of liver pyrrolase, the enzyme that degrades tryptophan.

If you can meditate, sun gaze, yoga and ground on the earth while "in the sun" it will help defrag your system so it can regain its circadian rhythm and homeostasis. The Inner Arts will really help, start out with the Heart-tree meditation, The Three Kings and Cardio Muscular Release to gain control over **the off-switch of your nervous system.** Primal Release Pose will relieve dis-ease and distress caught in your belly. Binaural music with ear phones or none will help. Try Alpha or the Awakening Mind Series 2 by Dr. Jeffrey Thompson Bio-Tuning® for sleep, stress, ADD, www.neuroacoustic.com/

• INSOMNIA HERBS

Herbs for calming nerves, insomnia, neuralgia, pain, shock, Die-off and depression of the down cycles, for tea, baths or capsulation: Syrian rue oil; Coptis Root, Horsemint or Bee Balm, Reishi, Catuaba bark, Borage, Burdock leaves, Chamomile, Catnip, Gorse flowers, California poppy flowers, Comfrey, Cowslip, Evening primrose, Ginger root, Goldenrod, Hop flowers, Juniper berries, Kava kava, Lemon balm, Linden flowers, Lobelia. Peppermint, Magnolia bark, Meadowsweet, Motherwort, Mulungu, Mullein, Nettle, Oatstraw, Passion flower, Red clover flowers, Rosemary leaf, Skullcap, St John's Wort, Valerian, Yarrow, Yellow dock. White willow and Wood Betony can be used as an anti-inflammatory for nerve pain and headaches.

• VISIONARY HERB MIX

Ashwagandha, Yerba mate, California Poppy, Magnolia bark, Mugwort, Angelica, Gotu Kola, Ginkgo, Borage, Rosemary, Ashitaba, Gorse Flowers, Nettle, Catnip, Horsetail, Diviner's Sage (Salvia divinorum), Rhodiola rosea root, Cayenne. Leave out the cayenne if you want to use this formula as a Tea.

These herbs (all parts) can be combined as either powders, essential oils or flower essences or taken as tea for increasing nerve coherence and psychic perception. They help to reintegrate and regenerate neurons, enhance neurocommunication, increase creativity, raise IQ, increase alpha and theta states, increase telepathy. Psychic and telepathic abilities are enhanced by increasing the sensitivity and coherency of individual nerve cells thereby stabilizing and integrating the instrument of consciousness. A good supply company is herbalcom.com

• SCENTS FOR SOVEREIGNTY

For perfume, anointing Oil and aromatherapy essential or absolute oils can be used to revive the senses, lift spirits and cleanse receptors. One of the best oils for sovereignty is blue lotus of Egypt, Nymphaea caerulea and Nelumbo nucifera (Sacred pink lotus). Genuine Lotus oil produces transcendence and transports us beyond everyday worries. Tuberose (Polianthes tuberosa), Ginger lily flower (Hedychium coranarium), the Gardenia (Gardenia jasminoides), or even the much richer, heavier scents of Kewda (Pandanus odoratissimus), Champaca (Michelia champaca), Plumeria (common name Frangipani). Datura oil an amazing sleep aid and dream enhancer, increasing the volume of dreams as well as the duration of dreams. The aromatic scent of magnolia (Michelia alba) promotes beauty, health, positivity and happiness.

• THE VISIONEER'S BATH

The same purification and enlivening practices one would use for raising kundalini will simultaneously increase the potential for visionary chemistry. Take a long, tall bath, preferably at least an hour long. Use Epsom salts in the bath, some essential oils, a candle, listen to heart stirring music. Drink 1-2 qts of water during the bath. Drop your tongue into your belly, do the inner smile and focus the mind's eye on your solar plexus. Put one hand over the right-side of the heart and the other on your solar plexus, breath into your solar plexus, empty your mind, feel into any pain or deficit you feel in your body. You may find the attention needs to be shifted to the thyroid throat area and the liver so put your hands over these, put your attention there and breathe into these areas.

The Visioneer's bath is useful both to increase the space and energy to invite visionary capacity, and for metabolizing and adjusting to extreme revelatory chemistry and ecstasy. Prolonged deep breathing in a float tank or bath, while clearing the mind and focusing all your energy and attention into the solar plexus (enteric brain), is a method of raising significant revelatory chemistry and for metabolizing, integrating and substantiating the "visions," so they can be bought into manifestation. These higher transpersonal, transrational layers of consciousness remain latent and impotent as long as we lack the strength of will, rational tenacity and heart to bring them into existence. Only we can green light our own spiritual-creative jeni and in doing so we raise ourselves towards the Divine.

The ancients had the benefit of closer planets, moon, sun etc... we socalled moderns however are more remote and dissociated, so lose out on a visceral gnostic knowledge of the music of the spheres. Plus our divorce from nature and her cycles reduces our senses and cosmic intelligence. Not to mention toxic EMF interference with the higher bands of human consciousness that key into the subtle frequencies of nature. Also our artificial lighting at night is one of the main blocks to a tacit relationship with the solar system and the stars, both visually, and by disrupting the circadian earth rhythms and Kairos or God's spiral time.

This loss of unification with the lunar, solar, planetary, circadian and Schumann resonances means that our melatonin/serotonin/DMT or spiritual chemistry is out of whack. In this way Borg consciousness, or the machine man can take ahold and we become prisoners of an unnatural culture. The sovereign HUman must find their way back to an energetic and cyclic reunion with Nature. As we unwind the Phi integrity inherent in the chiral perfection of natural order, the explosion technology civilization is winding its entropic way down to energy bankruptcy and oblivion.

The power-hungry imperialistic materialistic monopoly has been trying to wipe out personal sovereignty and immanent divine consciousness for over 2000 years, ever since the systematic extermination of the Gnostics and their direct knowledge of cosmic communion. By shunning a mystic view of the universe, humanity's moral compass that marries Mind, Matter and Spirit was lost. In a presovereign culture the individual feels subconsciously expendable and pressured to become prepersonal and self-sacrificing. As such their life is not their own and they are only as worthy as they are useful to others. Yet deep within the unlived recesses of our being we all know we have so much more to give than the world could ever receive.

Realizing the prison of unconscious conformity and knowing that love-mind can penetrate any darkness...we can find a way out of Borgsville to create a world that is workable, that makes sense, in which spirit can thrive as it wills. We free ourselves by turning inside for the answers and building up our latent capacities for Gnostic awareness or Grokking which have been kept from us over eons of disempowering cultural influence. Seeing through material reductionism and clearing away the ignorance of our painful past through philosophy, observation and self-inquiry we can bring on a cultural revolution of the Source directed life. The sovereign HUman is a Renaissance Man. Only mystic polymath geniuses are given sacred, secret access to nature's secrets through the sublime integration of body, mind and soul—tuned into the cosmos for the benefit of all life.

The Kin of Ata Are Waiting for You by Dorothy Bryant

Using Dreams and Creative Imagination for Personal Growth and Integration by Robert A. Johnson

APPENDIX B

SECRETS OF DAILY BLISS

There is no greater bliss than the ecstasy of aligning with the Force of Eros to bring about the birth of a genuine HUman being.

- **Increasing Painkilling Endorphins**—Things that increase endorphins: cayenne and jalapeño, raw greens, papaya smoothie, cayenne, rubbing or brushing the skin, bodywork, water therapy, alternating hot and cold, sunlight, exercise, stretching, hot and cold, positive thoughts, toning, humming, singing, meditating, deep breathing, music, pets, playing, nature's energies, waterfalls, the ocean, grounding, gardening, service to others, art, expression, truth, dropping the muscles at the back of the tongue and doing the Inner Smile etc....

- The increased neural activity of kundalini is associated with various degrees of bliss and ecstasy. This bliss is generated by opiates or endorphins, and the love chemicals including: nerve growth factor, testosterone, estrogen, dopamine, norepinephrine, serotonin, oxytocin, and vasopressin. The "molecule of love" phenylethylamine stimulates the brain to release a beta endorphin peptide that has analgesic effects and gives a feeling of well-being.

- Defensive "ego-armor" is the root-cause of our chronic resistance to the grace and the pleasure of life force.

- Spring water, hexagonal, structured, Vi-Aqua radio wave energised water, and high biogenic water provides the hydraulic matrix for bliss. www.viaqua.com

- A small spray bottle of ORMUS Cherokee trap water to spray on the neck (cherokeegold.net)—this allows the integration of bliss, basically making ecstasy easier to endure—perhaps by raising ATP production and creating a 8Hz the brain frequency for perfect phase conjunction

- Negative ions, grounding, moving water, sand, clay, nude dew baths on the lawn in the morning.

- I doubt you can have permanent bliss without a raw diet, so go mostly raw. Cooked food occludes the light and reduces the native bliss and joy of the body.

- Ultimately raw becomes imperative if you want to increasingly raise cell voltage and consciousness as everytime you eat cooked food or even boiled water you will notice a drop in consciousness. Raw living life cannot be fed on cooked dead food.

- Many will cling to their cannabis, antidepressants, sex, alcohol, power or danger — ultimately however these can never satisfy, for the only real, lasting bliss is the ecstasy of the sovereign presence.

• By blocking the light—sugar, alcohol, cigarettes and all processed and cooked food radically reduce the bliss of unity and enlightenment and diminish the body's capacity to love, hence the self-hatred and sadomasochism of the Borg.

• All that is alive and green: wheat grass, spirulina, dandelion greens, and sprouts keeps the bliss quotient up big time.

• Kelp, iodine, DHEA–morning and Melatonin-evening act to deeply recharge and relax.

• The beta carotene in Papaya smoothies and living Hawaii generates bliss.

• Adaptogenic herbs like Ashitaba, Ashwaganda, Ginseng, Rhodiola rosa, Maral root and Dong quai.

• Bliss herbs include Ashwagandha, Basil, Banisteriopsis caapi, California poppy, Cayenne, Codonopsis, Corydalis elata, Angelica, Gorse flowers, Passionflower, Muira Puama, Maca, Mucuna pruriens.

• By mixing Mucuna, Caapi and Gingko and taking around: 2 x 000 capsules I was able to integrate the bliss trance of kundalini, come out of brain fog and achieve a newfound lucidity. So this may be due to boosting dopamine and reducing the serotonin overload which normally goes along with bliss-heat-fluxes. Thus we can have our bliss and our lucidity too.

• Becoming a herb shaman and taking lots of medicinal and culinary herbs and wild plants in teas, capsules, baths and with meals sustains your bliss potential. A phytochemical rich diet is essential for bliss and the reduction of entropy.

• Syrian rue-Galangal-Ginger tincture increases serotonin and improves circulation, allowing a profound settling, relaxation and heart expansion. Increases coordination between the head-heart-stomach brains, and promotes dreaming if used at night.

• Strong chamomile tea infusion heated on low heat and filtered, then put into a spray bottle to spray all over the body and hair…raises immunity and reduces body pain.

• Spark up your kundalini by raising cell voltage and communication by reducing acid pH in body with fresh vegetable juice and green smoothies.

• Get plenty of aerobic exercise in the fresh air and sun, essential to keeping the flows going for bliss. Bliss requires a clean, well-hydrated and well-oxygenated temple.

• Any form of light, sound, vibration, movement or massage to get the lymphatic system going increases bliss.

• Bliss requires happy organs and clean lymph so rebound as the sun rises.

• If you fall out of bliss go for a 4 hour breath-walk to recharge.

- Sungazing at dawn/dusk builds blissful plasma in the brain that lasts for days.

- Sunbathing and increasing vitamin D reenergizes hormones and energy levels and removes pain. Ecstasy requires the sun to produce Vitamin D and catalyze mineral use for the superconducting state of bliss.

- Humming, singing, toning (HU) greatly enhances daily bliss.

- All the Inner Arts and kundalini exercises generate bliss.

- Following your bliss, the Muse and your soul vocation greatly increases bliss by reducing conflicting motivations and creating spiritual alignment. Ultimately this is the maximum bliss path.

- Hot and cold or anything that gets your circulation going and blood oxygenated is good for bliss.

- To conserve energy you may need to reduce sex or masturbation down to once a month if over 45, but then you are usually too blissed out to want it anyway.

- Grounding on the ground, going barefoot, clay inside and out, fasting, detoxifying practices like saunas, steam rooms, bodywork, body brushing.

- Giving away things you no longer need generates bliss, but it can be addictive if it stems from the need for approval. It is best to focus on your muse and giving your greatest gift than becoming distracted by lower order giving that does nothing to uplift the state of mankind.

- Our love in action is who we become. Basically doing what you love, and looking after your bodymind, cultivating friends, remembering the dream and having determination to keep the greater.

- What you use to accelerate the growth of your abilities, IS your abilities.

- Every moment of fear blocks our awareness of love's presence, while discovering the adventure of being alive generates all the bliss you will ever need.

- The high of Mystical writers must be one of the bests drugs on earth — dozens of times while writing BOK I was in extreme ecstasy, awe and excitement. Such illuminating chemistry couldn't be achieved by any other means. Original thought, gnosis, eurekas, revelation, mystical level thought comes from such a liberated place that it elevates us completely out of the mundane humdrum world and into a scintillating enchanted kingdom. Visions and dreams have a similar enchanting quality if they are of the transcendental level. Falling in love can also produce this magic quality of indescribably bliss that lifts us beyond the known.

- ReNature First—The body is trying to normalize, or rather optimize itself, and cannot do so without nature's energies. Engage in meditative, healing and exercise practices in nature on the grass, rocks, beach or water. If you are not using Nature's energies forget trying to optimize or normalize cause it an't going to happen.

- You can't be well when you are focusing on feeling awful. Make yourself feel good, relaxed, happy, complete, blissful, connected, loved, groovy, valuable NOW!

Understanding and Activating Your Brain's Pleasure Centers ~ Jonathan Cowan, Ph.D. and John Starman, MA

PLAYFUL CONCLUSION

"We either make ourselves miserable or we make ourselves strong. The amount of work is the same." Carlos Castaneda

To give birth to the future requires the realization of sovereignty as the source code of our salvation and our reason for being. We are collectively moving toward being able to visualize that which we actually WANT and have the sovereign potency to bring it about. To actualize what we want we must envision our desired goal and see it as complete, whole and finished. Through time and synchronicity we then step into and appreciate the vision as if it were always already here. Paradoxically, the more we let go, the more things seemed to take off. Once you enter the sovereign path there is such a resurgence of hope, because we relax into the proficiency of cocreativity. As we merge with cosmic Flow, Spirit reveals to us exactly the next nuanced piece of the puzzle toward transcendental freedom.

Befriending and embracing our sovereign Self on the deepest embodied level permits us to operate from the fullness paradigm through "trust in the heart's cosmic intelligence." It actually takes a lot of work to make ourselves miserable, and a lot of play to make ourselves strong. Learning to play is the true work. Unlicensed, unlimited and unabashed PLAY is always the solution to everything. Finding ever higher forms of play is the spiritual quest. If our work becomes play we can achieve the excellence of the genius of the Universe pouring through us. A lavish exuberant sense of play and the consequent reduction in fear and anxiety, increases higher brain function and purifies negativities. Divine play is both the vehicle and the destination. The art of love is Divine Play!

"It is a widely held view that the animal that plays - or practices - will become more expert, and thereby have a selective advantage over the animal that does not." 184, Primate Ethology, Desmond Morris

APPENDIX C

TENETS OF DIVINE PLAY

- **Integration**—Divine play leads to the evolution of our self-awareness…that is being conscious that we are conscious. Greater integration means greater integrity, and a synchronization of the parts to establish a more cohesive whole. As we learn to better Know Thyself we can up grade our living dream more to our personal choosing

- **Resistance is the Key** — The divine mind is not the ego…the defensive ego armoring is "resistance" to the divine consciousness which we have yet to realize as a human being. Resistance to dysfunction is a trap that keeps us from knowledge of our Self. Therefore our resistance to acknowledgement of our dynsfunction the Key to the unveiling of the Self.

- **Transformation** — Transcendence prior to transformation is dissociation, which presents itself as addiction, illness, codependency, crime, plus unconscious and compulsive behaviors that lead to greater life challenges. True transcendence (ie: freedom) is acquired through transformation in working through and mastering life challenges as they arise.

- **A Priori Causal State**—Recognition of our fundamental Self-responsibility is paramount. You are the cause of your feelings, thoughts and emotions. Awareness of self-origination is the heart of mindfulness.

- **Wakefulness** — Mindfulness is how you maintain the vital edge of your daily play and prevent the contagion of unhappy thoughts and experiences. Self-regulate by using the world as a mirror for your own emotional tone.

- **Good-Will**—First do no harm is a basic rule of divine play that goes along with the Golden Rule. Do no harm in thought, word or deed and you up-spiral your energy and love.

- **Open-Ended Desire**—Wish for the "best outcome ever" rather than sticking to a tight action plan, for we cannot anticipate the exact course of events and must remain open to the changing hologram of the unfolding world.

- **Equanimity** — If the metamorphic process proceeds with adequate grace, then the Percival Heart is born, or the Heart that is radiant and open irrespective of external conditions.

- **Nonduality** — Follow your heart! The Percival or Open Heart is your navigator. Thus your compass must be unguarded, void of paranoia, soft, furry and good-willing in order to meet its happy mark. However, when you're swimming in the ocean and you see a shark approaching get out of the water.

- **Cultural Debriefing** — When emerging beyond veil of conditioning we can use an intensive interview format with a fair witness to objectively run through our life story through the eyes of an anthropological myth. This acts as a psychic laxative and brings cohesion and wholeness to our sense of well-being.

- **Molting** — Off load all that is keeping you from the vital edge of divine play so you can accumulate momentum and keep pace with the speed of spirit's evolution.

- **Transform Fear** — Use fear as a heat seeking missile to the realization of courage. As we make proactive steps that transcend our fear rather than react to it, we feel courage, power and exhilaration.

- **Choice** — You get to play whatever role in whatever movie you want. You get to write and direct your movie; plus you are the financier and the audience…so enjoy because it is "your" movie!

- **Ascension** — In moving out of victimhood (its all done to me) we must realize our role in the creation of "difficulty" and work to change our energy to up-spiral creative director of our lives.

- **Clarity** — By adopting a clear perspective and courageous outlook on the situation, you will be better prepared to survive even the longest battle, regardless of the ongoing successes and failures, or the ultimate result.

- **Veil of Perception** — Our lens of perception (energetic state) is more important than perceived circumstances, thus we must fast, run, get bodywork, meditate, do Inner Arts, yoga, climb a mountain etc to reinstate our evolutionary (up-spiral) energy.

- **Embrace Reality** — Difficulty presents the greatest growth opportunity. Nothing is insurmountable if we approach it in positive-play and without fear…continually learning and creating within the hologram.

- **Beginner's Mind** — To keep a plastic brain, we must realize the plastic nature of reality and yield not to recursive habit, but turn towards the spontaneous joyous unfoldment of creation.

- **Vigor of the New** — By becoming a novelty seeker we continue to learn throughout our lives and remain young and innocent at heart. Divine Play is the elixir of youth.

- **Self as Source** — Fill up on your own love first, for seeking to be fed from the world while in the deprivation state just makes us more hungry, lost and bereft of meaning. We can never be satisfied by the world without first establishing the organic satisfaction of being in our own body.

- **Nirvana Now** — At all times Universe is conspiring to awaken us to unity consciousness. So we might as well surrender to Nirvana Now, for Nirvana can only be known Now, regardless of where or how we find ourselves.

- **Patience** — As we accumulate the momentum of divine play we need understanding and patience when encountering the "time lag" in actually manifesting a changed life from our changed beliefs and new intentions. Material reality seems like eons behind mystical reality, hence patience is in order.

• **Take Charge**—Claim full responsibility for social interactions, not because everything is "your fault" but because this empowers you to change your energy state, attitude and circumstances. If you are always blaming the other guy for being mad and unreasonable, then you will not be able to focus on doing what it takes to develop lubricated social ease and raise your energy and social power.

• **Containment**—Indiscriminate "teaching" to those in the consensus trance generates friction, for many people are too stressed, sick and conservative to tolerate enlightening words beyond the given matrix. Thus we must establish our own peer forums, salons, workshops and venues for expression without necessarily taking it to the streets.

• **Be the Teaching**—First and foremost we must build up our own physical, emotional, mental and psychic strength and quit trying to enlighten, teach heal and save a world. If we BE the example in time, the world automatically shifts to the higher vibration without us having to force it into existence.

• **Harvest of Dreams**—Sleep is the highest consciousness period, for we get our deepest information and integration and precognition while sleeping... hence our pre-bed practice needs to include stretches, spinal rolling, breathing, water, music in order to set the stage for higher conscious visionary sleep.

• **Curiosity**—Any animal in seeking mode has active dopamine circuits and can feel the Flow of Eros directing and inspiring their actions. Alpha frequency tunes animals into the "planetary vibe and wholebrain integration," where curiosity and anticipation arise simultaneously with novelty, synchronicity, surprise and fascination with the unknown. The world of the sovereign therefore with lush dopamine dendrites is an expression of Eros rather than the default programming of Thanatos given to us by the death culture, which is defeated before it even begins.

• **Observation** — Significance and meaning perceived from inquisitive contact with nature's harmonies and extensive interconnections, leads to the revitalization of empathy and involvement in both inner, inter and intra human relationships.

• **Adventure**—Through adventure we find our edge and put ourselves in various new and risky situations that quicken our spiritual metabolism. Adventure means facing challenge and so real life skills are learnt. Thus we evolve by living out our hero's journey.

• **Celebration**—The old must die for the new to be reborn, hence the highs and lows of happenstance should be celebrated equally. The art of play celebrates and savors the intricate flavors of all experience as the fastest route beyond the prison of self-centric ego.

- **Fun Magnet** — Establishing the frequency of divine play, we induce the accumulation and acceleration of fun and personal magnetism. As our magnetism for fun increases we draw to us humor, synchronicity, fun, play and happiness and we spread it in equal measure. This serendipity is the alchemical born of unity.

- **Flow** — Appreciation and gratitude is the key to transformation. For we cannot transform that which we are rebelling, repulsing or resisting. With the expansiveness of appreciation we flow like water around the stones in the river of life.

- **Upping The Game** — We can withdraw, transcend and up our game at any point…by zeroing out of the existing play mode through Attraction Meditation, Sun Gazing, Spinal Shower, Binaural Theta Wave, Grounding etc… By becoming more lucid we can then find and embody the higher conscious solution to current drama.

- **Detachment** — Detachment with full empathetic understanding is the highest power for full embodiment, dispassionate objectivity and fearlessness. If we are immune to attachment and possession then nothing will possess us. He who is master of his possessions, rather than being possessed by them is the wise master of his universe.

- **Attraction = Radiance** — The keys to the Law of Attraction are: "you achieve what you believe;" "what you focus on expands;" and "the flipside of attraction is contribution." That is you get what you want by giving others what they want.

- **The Law of Attraction** — We attract into our experience that with which vibrationally resonates with our thoughts and feelings. We mistakenly think that we feel the way we do BECAUSE of our circumstances, when in fact our circumstances are a reflection of the way we feel.

- **Discernment** — You CAN have it all. This requires faith and belief. It also requires that you stop spending your precious time on things of little inherent value to you, and start pursuing what really matters.

- **Believing** — The more we stay in touch with the rewarding positive feelings that each goal delivers, especially in our imagination, the more motivated and committed we'll be to continue the pursuit. Anticipation produces dopamine as a "reward' chemical in the brain which motivates and energizes you. Believe you can succeed and you will.

- **Receiving** — You can't appreciate what you take for granted. Therefore appreciation or gratitude is the key to happiness. If you are not grateful for what you have chances are you will not appreciate getting "more" either.

- **Radiant Enlightenment** — The empowered, enfranchised, sovereign HUman finds enlightenment, entertainment, purpose, meaning and joy inside themselves. Our mystical, magical divine Self is always already a part of us.

RESOURCES

- www.neuroacoustic.com — Dr. Jeffrey Thompson binaural brainwave music
- Fabrication Enterprises Cando Inflatable Roller 7″ x 17″ is a cylinder exercise roller-ball for dearmoring via spinal rolling.
- Tennis balls are good for rolling your back on and self-massaging on the floor.
- *Stress: Portrait of a Killer* — Learn how social stress is the most pernicious and pervasive form of stress watch Robert Sapolsky's documentary DVD and lectures on youtube.
- *Bouncing Back: Rewiring Your Brain for Maximum Resilience and Well-Being*, by Linda Graham and Rick Hanson. An ideal companion to The Inner Arts. http://www.kickbully.com — Fantastic site for dealing with bullies.
- *The Shamanic Odyssey: Homer, Tolkien, and the Visionary Experience*, Robert Tindall. Important book about Shamanic initiation, addiction, and cultivating the indigenous mind.
- LED LIGHT CRYSTAL WAND — You can make a quartz crystal LED torch wand to use in healing that heals the healer as they heal. You get a little LED torch from army surplus then put a flat bottom round topped crystal wand in a plastic bottle lid by carving a hole in it, then fit it on the torch with plastic tape. This makes a light-lit-quartz-wand with a friendly warm vibe. Acculightpressure increases biophotons in areas that need to energize, wake up and decontract in order to heal. Ideally the crystal should not be too pointy but rounded, (you can get good ones from ebay)…and you can have a series of different kinds of transparent crystals. Applied to the jaw, temple, neck, pineal gland the light energy loosens tissue and generates bliss and vitality in the area. The light wand can be used on the acupuncture points, joints, thymus or sluggish organs and anywhere there are areas of tightness, congestion and pain in the body. Use it to energize the body's meridians by applying the wand to the fascia system. The lit wand can also be held over the thymus gland on the chest in The Light Sword Meditation. You can fit this wand into a hole cut into a bottle lid and use it to charge your drinking water.
- BINAURAL MUSIC like Jeffery Thompson's www.neuroacoustic.com or Willy Smith www.WillFortune.com. Bi-frequency enables the synchronization or binaural beating of the hemispheres of the brain. This effect underlies the ancient Sanskrit kundalini tradition and technology that originated in the antediluvian mother-culture of Atlantis.
- GAMA FREQUENCY — activates DNA expression. All of Jeffrey Thompson's CDs including "Gamma Meditation" are extremely effective at inducing meditative states. Thompson is a pioneer in brainwave entrainment research, and is the one who discovered Epsilon waves (slower than Delta, less than 1/2 Hz per second), among other things.
- SOUND OF THE SUN — David Sereda's 7 minute CD on the sound of the sun for charging our water can be purchased through his website www.voiceentertainment.net
- 528 Hz is the Solfeggio frequency used by biochemists to repair DNA!

http://www.sourcevibrations.com/ —Sacred geometric sound design, integrating golden mean mathematics, universal harmonics, and Solfeggio frequencies to establish resonant fields of internal coherence.
• www.cessulta.com — Cranial Electrotherapy Stimulator (CES) good for increasing the plasticity of the nervous system to allow change in response to ones sovereignty/awakening practice.
• www.pulsedharmonix.com — Pulsed Electromanetic Field Therapy
• Conair-Body-Rhythms-Massager — If you get this particular massager you can lie on it and massage your adrenals, kidneys back, feet etc... Massaging the adrenals will reduce inflammation, allergies, over-active immune system, sinus, liver and kidney detox, etc....It has two pulsating rubber nodes that provide a unique tapping pulsation.
• http://omgym.com/ —Aerial Yoga Swing to radically open up body armor.
• www.aircat.net/Aerial/Equipment.html —Aerial Yoga Silk and hardware
Nutrition Supplies:
www.herbalcom.com — Best site for inexpensive herb supplies and clay etc.
https://herbprod.com — Herbal Products and Development nutrition supplies
www.Beyond-a-Century.com — Great supplement supply company
www.swansonsvitamins.com — Inexpensive supplements
www.mountainroseherbs.com — Great comprehensive selection
http://www.organicfruitsandnuts.com — Jaffe Bros., Inc. Seeds and nuts
http://thesyncbook.com/ —Synchronicity exploration community and books

HYDROGENATED WATER: Hydrogen-rich water is antioxidant, anti-aging, boosts metabolism, reduces fatigue and improves mood. As hydrogen is the smallest element in the universe, it easily penetrates the entire body, including the neurons and the cell nuclei. Hydrogen increases the pH of water by half a point to 7 or 7.5, combating the acidity that results from toxicity, inflammation and oxidation in the body. To purchase a **Hydrogenizer Bottle** with Titanium electrodes to avoid heavy metal poisoning email **H2@wingscoaching.com**

THE EMANCIPATOR and THE SPINAL ROLLER
Emancipation Unlimited LLC
If you are an international ecommerce entrepreneur looking for a new product contact me for the ultimate fun e-enterprise. jananz@hotmail.com

www.biologyofkundalini.com
http://jana-sovereignstate.blogspot.com
https://biologyofkundalini.academia.edu/JanaDixon

***More on neurobiology of personal sovereignty in upcoming books in the Awakening Sovereignty series.

BIBLIOGRAPHY

Orgone, Reich and Eros, by W. Edward Mann
The Emotional Plague: The Root of Human Evil, by Charles Konia
Dismantling Contemporary Deficit Thinking: Educational Thought and Practice, by Richard R. Valencia
Energy Medicine; the Scientific Basis, by James Oschman
Janus: A Summing Up, Arthur Koestler
The Empathic Civilization: The Race to Global Consciousness in a World in Crisis, by Jeremy Rifkin
The Bond: Connecting Through the Space Between Us, by Lynne McTaggart
The Human Antenna: Reading the Language of the Universe in the Songs of Our Cells, by Dr Robin Kelly
Seeds for Another World, by Florin Munteanu
The Power of Limits, by Gyorgy Doczi
The Secret of Light, by Walter Russell
Untethered Soul, by Michael A. Singer
The Presence Process: A Healing Journey into Present Moment Awareness, by Michael Brown
Emotional Intimacy: A Comprehensive Guide for Connection with the Power of Emotions, by Robert Augustus Masters
Emotional Life of Your Brain, by Richard J. Davidson
Incognito: The Secret Lives of the Brain, by David Eagleman
Mirroring People: The Science of Empathy and How We Connect with Others, by Marco Iacoboni
The Eight-Circuit Brain: Navigational Strategies for the Energetic Body, Antero Alli
Power Up Your Brain: The Neuroscience of Enlightenment, by David Perlmutter MD and Alberto Villoldo Ph.D.
Happiness Genes: Unlock the Positive Potential Hidden in Your DNA, by James Baird, Laurie Nadel and Bruce Lipton
Left in the Dark: The Biological Origins of the Fall From Grace, by Tony Wright
The Betrayal of the Body; and *Narcissism: Denial of the True Self*, by Alexander Lowen
Focusing, by Eugene Gendlin
Emotional Wisdom: Daily Tools for Transforming Anger, Depression, and Fear, by Mantak Chia
The Self Illusion: How the Social Brain Creates Identity, by Bruce Hood
How to Thrive in Changing Times, by Sandra Igerman
Tales of the San Francisco Cacophony Society is a valuable book for generating more fun, authenticity and spontaneity in your life, along the lines of *The Diceman*, by Luke Reinhart
The Televisionary Oracle, by Rob Brezsny
See: David Wolfe's Earthing Experiment on youtube
www.longevitywarehouse.com — David Wolfe's website
The Vivaxis Connection: Healing Through Earth Energies by Judy Jacka

Earthing: The Most Important Health Discovery Ever? by Clinton Ober, Stephen T. Sinatra, and Martin Zucker
www.earthing.com/ sell grounding sheets and mats
www.gelearthing.com — Earthing Supply Company
www.lessemf.com/ground.html — Grounding Equipment
Boiling Energy: Community Healing Among the Kalahari Kung by Richard Katz
www.bradfordkeeny.com.br — *Bushman Shaman: Awakening the Spirit through Ecstatic Dance* by Bradford Keeney
Ceramic Houses - Earth Architecture: How to Build Your Own, by Nader Khalili
See Youtube Video: *Jon Young Speaks About The Role of Deep Nature Connection in Culture Repair*

ADVANCED MEDIA
www.brighteon.com — Video Media Sans The Thought Police
www.redicecreations.com — Henrik Palmgren, Favorite interview site
www.freedomainradio.com/Podcasts.aspx — Stefan Molyneux podcasts
https://futurethinkers.org/jordan-greenhall-deep-code — Jordan-Greenhall
https://neurohacker.com/collective_insights_podcast — Uplifting
thecrowhouse.com — Max Igan, Spiritual Father on equity.
http://legalise-freedom.com — Greg Moffitt, Legalise Freedom radio
www.enigmatv.com — Christopher Everard, Very comprehensive thinker
www.neilkramer.com — Neil Kramer, Earthsoul development
http://whatonearthishappening.com — Mark Passio, Natural Law
http://sovereignman.com — Simon Black, Global citizen newsletters
www.progressiveradionetwork.com — Dr. Gary Null and other hosts!
https://www.darkjournalist.com/— Daniel Liszt independent reporter
prn.fm/category/archives/expanding-mind — Erik Davis, Expanding Mind
www.tragedyandhope.com — Richard Grove, Metaview Affairs
http://educate-yourself.org — Freedom Information Hub
www.nexusmagazine.com — Building the New World
www.wordpress.peakmoment.tv/conversations/ — Post Carbon TV
www.hiddenincatours.com — Brien Foerster, Coneheads, Tours, Books
http://slavespecies.com — Michael Tellinger, Ancient S.Africa, UBUNTU
www.philosophy.org — Walter Russell, True Cosmological science
www.thrivemovement.com — Foster Gamble, Community growth network
globalbem.com — Breakthrough Energy Movement
http://peswiki.com — New Energy Info Nexus and Achives
www.rts.earth — Removing the Shackles, Transpicuous News
Pocketnet.app — Pocketnet is a fully decentralized publishing and social platform., based on the blockchain technology.

For **Grand Solar Minimum Preparedness** keep up with Youtube Channels: Adapt 2030, Ice Age Farmer, the Grand Solar Minimum channel, Oppenheimer Ranch, Suspicious0bservers, ThunderboltsProject and John Casey.

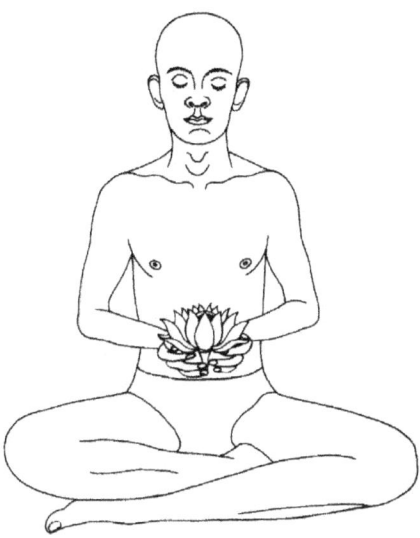

Everything humanity does to try and save itself within the power hunger of the presovereign Borg zeitgeist will only precipitate a faster decline. It is obvious therefore that what is needed is a revolution of the heart and mind, leading to the reimagining of what it is to be HUman. Abundance is the natural state of growth achieved through sharing, respect, synergy, generosity, over-utility, creativity, magnanimity, faith, interest, engagement and goodwill. An enlightened civilization is founded on the principles of cosmic abundance.

There is the "divine grace" aspect of creative expression, the receiving, which we normally only get if we have been obedient to the directives of our assigned sacred duty. Then there is the "effort-work-practice" needed to raise our mortal bodymind up to the holy condition through which we can be a sublime vehicle for the execution of our assigned sacred duty.

This transpersonal illumination is visited upon us from a realm that is beyond our regular conditioned senses and perception of the world. The sacred "Muse" is beyond time and space and so there is no barrier to the gnostic knowledge that we can "receive" through enchanted visions, dreams, precognition, telepathy, voices, and psychic senses and sublime emotions.

Such sacred creativity is the way of the future, and the way into the transcendental future we know in our hearts is possible.

www.ingramcontent.com/pod-product-compliance
Lightning Source LLC
Chambersburg PA
CBHW062220080426
42734CB00010B/1967